SESSION	TOPIC	CONTENTS

ACKNOWLEDGEMENTS

Radcliffe Medical Press acknowledges with gratitude the kind permission granted by publishers of the citation references for the full papers to be reproduced at the beginning of each session. These permissions prohibit further reproduction by photocopying or by electronic means and if this facility is required, further permission should be obtained from the source quoted in each case.

Extracts from *Evidence-based Medicine: how to practice and teach EBM* (David Sackett *et al.*) which appear at the back of this manual are reproduced with the kind permission of Harcourt Brace & Co Ltd.

This is a syllabus for a 7 session course for clinicians on how to practice evidence-based medicine: that is, how to integrate our individual clinical expertise with a critical appraisal of the best available external clinical evidence from systematic research.

We see the practice of evidence-based medicine as a process of life-long, self-directed, problem based learning in which caring for one's own patients creates the need for clinically important information about diagnosis, prognosis, therapy, and other clinical and health care issues, in which its practitioners:

1   convert these information needs into answerable questions;

2   track down, with maximum efficiency, the best evidence with which to answer them (making best use of the increasing variety of sources of primary and secondary evidence);

3   critically appraise that evidence for its validity (closeness to the truth) importance (size of effect) and usefulness (clinical applicability);

4   integrate the appraisal with clinical expertise and apply the results in clinical practice; and

5   evaluate their own performance.

This syllabus is designed to help clinicians develop and improve those skills. In addition, it is designed to help Membership candidates prepare for the EBM portions of the Membership Examination.

Each of its 7 sessions is divided into 2 parts:

Part A: Going through the 5 steps with a patient, focusing on step 3 (critical appraisal), step 4 (integration with clinical expertise), and step 5 (self-evaluation).

Part B: Skills training, focusing on step 1 (forming answerable clinical questions) and step 2 (finding the best evidence), in which we introduce a variety of sources of evidence plus some strategies for analysing, summarising and storing the evidence in the form of one-page summaries ("Critically Appraised Topics" or CATs).

Evidence-based Medicine: what it is and what it isn't

This is the text of an editorial from the *British Medical Journal* of 13th January 1996 (*BMJ* 1996; **312**: 71–2)

Authors:

David L Sackett, Professor, NHS Research and Development Centre for Evidence-based Medicine, Oxford.

William MC Rosenberg, Clinical Tutor in Medicine, Nuffield Department of Clinical Medicine, Oxford.

JA Muir Gray, Director of Research and Development, Anglia and Oxford Regional Health Authority, Milton Keynes

R Brian Haynes, Professor of Medicine and Clinical Epidemiology, McMaster University Hamilton, Canada

W Scott Richardson, Rochester, USA

Evidence-based medicine, whose philosophical origins extend back to mid-19th century Paris and earlier, remains a hot topic for clinicians, public health practitioners, purchasers, planners and the public. There are now frequent workshops in how to practice and teach it (one sponsored by this journal will be held in London on April 24th); undergraduate [1] and post-graduate training programmes [2] are incorporating it [3] (or pondering how to do so); British centres for evidence-based practice have been established or planned in adult medicine, child health, surgery, pathology, pharmacotherapy, nursing, general practice, and dentistry; the Cochrane Collaboration and the York Centre for Review and Dissemination in York are providing systematic reviews of the effects of health care; new evidence-based practice journals are being launched; and it has become a common topic in the lay media. But enthusiasm has been mixed with some negative reaction [4–6]. Criticism has ranged from evidence-based medicine being old-hat to it being a dangerous innovation, perpetrated by the arrogant to serve cost-cutters and suppress clinical freedom. As evidence-based medicine continues to evolve and adapt, now is a useful time to refine the discussion of what it is and what it is not.

Evidence-based medicine is the conscientious, explicit and judicious use of current best evidence in making decisions about the care of individual patients. The practice of evidence-based medicine means integrating individual clinical expertise with the best available external clinical evidence from systematic research. By individual clinical expertise we mean the proficiency and judgement that individual clinicians acquire through clinical experience and clinical practice. Increased expertise is reflected in many ways, but especially in more effective and efficient diagnosis and in the more thoughtful identification and compassionate use of individual patients' predicaments, rights, and preferences in making clinical decisions about their care. By best available external clinical evidence we mean clinically relevant research, often from the basic sciences of medicine, but especially from patient centred clinical research into the accuracy and precision of diagnostic tests (including the clinical examination), the power of prognostic markers, and the efficacy and safety of therapeutic, rehabilitative, and preventive regimens. External clinical evidence both invalidates previously accepted diagnostic tests and treatments and replaces them with new ones that are more powerful, more accurate, more efficacious, and safer.

Good doctors use both individual clinical expertise and the best available external evidence, and neither alone is enough. Without clinical expertise, practice risks becoming tyrannised by evidence, for even excellent external evidence may be inapplicable to or inappropriate for an individual patient. Without current best evidence, practice risks becoming rapidly out of date, to the detriment of patients.

This description of what evidence-based medicine is helps clarify what evidence-based medicine is not. Evidence-based medicine is neither old-hat nor impossible to practice. The argument that everyone already is doing it falls before evidence of striking variations in both the integration of patient values into our clinical behaviour [7] and in the rates with which clinicians provide interventions to their patients [8]. The difficulties that clinicians face in keeping abreast of all the medical advances reported in primary journals are obvious from a comparison of the time required for reading (for general medicine, enough to examine

19 articles per day, 365 days per year [9]) with the time available (well under an hour per week by British medical consultants, even on self-reports [10]).

The argument that evidence-based medicine can be conducted only from ivory towers and armchairs is refuted by audits in the front lines of clinical care where at least some inpatient clinical teams in general medicine [11], psychiatry (JR Geddes, *et al*, Royal College of Psychiatrists winter meeting, January 1996), and surgery (P McCulloch, personal communication) have provided evidence-based care to the vast majority of their patients. Such studies show that busy clinicians who devote their scarce reading time to selective, efficient, patient-driven searching, appraisal and incorporation of the best available evidence can practice evidence-based medicine.

Evidence-based medicine is not "cook-book" medicine. Because it requires a bottom-up approach that integrates the best external evidence with individual clinical expertise and patient-choice, it cannot result in slavish, cook-book approaches to individual patient care. External clinical evidence can inform, but can never replace, individual clinical expertise, and it is this expertise that decides whether the external evidence applies to the individual patient at all and, if so, how it should be integrated into a clinical decision. Similarly, any external guideline must be integrated with individual clinical expertise in deciding whether and how it matches the patient's clinical state, predicament, and preferences, and thus whether it should be applied. Clinicians who fear top-down cook-books will find the advocates of evidence-based medicine joining them at the barricades.

Evidence-based medicine is not cost-cutting medicine. Some fear that evidence-based medicine will be hijacked by purchasers and managers to cut the costs of health care. This would not only be a misuse of evidence-based medicine but suggests a fundamental misunderstanding of its financial consequences. Doctors practising evidence-based medicine will identify and apply the most efficacious interventions to maximise the quality and quantity of life for individual patients; this may raise rather than lower the cost of their care.

Evidence-based medicine is not restricted to randomised trials and meta-analyses. It involves tracking down the best external evidence with which to answer our clinical questions. To find out about the accuracy of a diagnostic test, we need to find proper cross-sectional studies of patients clinically suspected of harbouring the relevant disorder, not a randomised trial. For a question about prognosis, we need proper follow-up studies of patients assembled at a uniform, early point in the clinical course of their disease. And sometimes the evidence we need will come from the basic sciences such as genetics or immunology. It is when asking questions about therapy that we should try to avoid the non-experimental approaches, since these routinely lead to false-positive conclusions about efficacy. Because the randomised trial, and especially the systematic review of several randomised trials, is so much more likely to inform us and so much less likely to mislead us, it has become the "gold standard" for judging whether a treatment does more good than harm. However, some questions about therapy do not require randomised trials (successful interventions for otherwise fatal conditions) or cannot wait for the trials to be conducted. And if no randomised trial has been carried out for our patient's predicament, we follow the trail to the next best external evidence and work from there.

Despite its ancient origins, evidence-based medicine remains a relatively young discipline whose positive impacts are just beginning to be validated [12, 13], and it will continue to evolve. This evolution will be enhanced as several undergraduate, post-graduate, and continuing medical education programmes adopt and adapt it to their learners' needs. These programmes, and their evaluation, will provide further information and understanding about what evidence-based medicine is, and what it is not.

References

1 British Medical Association: *Report of the working party on medical education*. London: British Medical Association, 1995.

2 Standing Committee on Postgraduate Medical and Dental Education: *Creating a better learning environment in hospitals: 1 Teaching hospital doctors and dentists to teach*. London: SCOPME, 1994.

3 General Medical Council: *Education Committee Report*. London: General Medical Council, 1994.

4 Grahame-Smith D: Evidence-based medicine: Socratic dissent. *BMJ* 1995; 310:1126–7.

5 Evidence-based medicine, in its place (editorial). *Lancet* 1995; 346:785.

6 Correspondence. Evidence-based Medicine. *Lancet* 1995; 346:1171–2

7 Weatherall DJ: The inhumanity of medicine. *BMJ* 1994; 308:1671–2.

8 House of Commons Health Committee. *Priority setting in the NHS: purchasing*. First report sessions 1994–95. London: HMSO, 1995, (HC 134–1.)

9 Davidoff F, Haynes B, Sackett D, Smith R: Evidence-based medicine; a new journal to help doctors identify the information they need. *BMJ* 1995; 310:1085–6.

10 Sackett DL: Surveys of self-reported reading times of consultants in Oxford, Birmingham, Milton-Keynes, Bristol, Leicester, and Glasgow, 1995. In Rosenberg WMC, Richardson WS, Haynes RB, Sackett DL. *Evidence-based Medicine*. London: Churchill-Livingstone, 1999.

11 Ellis J, Mulligan I, Rowe J, Sackett DL: Inpatient general medicine is evidence based. *Lancet* 1995; 346:407–10.

12 Bennett RJ, Sackett DL, Haynes RB, Neufeld VR: A controlled trial of teaching critical appraisal of the clinical literature to medical students. *JAMA* 1987; 257: 2451–4.

13 Shin JH, Haynes RB, Johnston ME: Effect of problem-based, self-directed undergraduate education on life-long learning. *Can Med Assoc J* 1993;148:969–76.

Introduction

PART

A **Critical appraisal of a clinical article about therapy**

You see a 72-year old man referred to you by his GP with sudden onset of left-sided weakness and numbness, and a left homonymous hemianopia. His past medical history is unremark-able and he is not on any medications. On physical exam he has improved but still has evidence of moderate left-sided weakness consistent with MCA territory stroke; he also has a right carotid bruit. His GP had told him about an operation that could 'clean' his arteries out and wanted to know if this could be done. You aren't sure, and form the clinical question: 'In patients with a recent cerebrovascular event and high-grade stenosis of the ipsilateral internal carotid artery, does carotid endarterectomy reduce the risk of subsequent major stroke and death?'

You start up *Best Evidence*, enter 'carotid endarterectomy,' and you find the abstract for the randomised trial of endarterectomy in patients with symptomatic high-grade stenosis from the New England Journal report of the North American Symptomatic Carotid Endarterectomy Trial. The abstract and commentary look very promising, so you go to the library and copy the original article: (*N Engl J Med* (1991) **325**: 445–53).[1]

Read this article and decide:
1   Is the evidence from this randomised trial valid?
2   If valid, is this evidence important?
3   If valid and important, **and if your patient was shown to have an appropriate carotid lesion**, can you apply this evidence in caring for your patient?

(If you want to read some strategies for answering these sorts of questions, look at pp 91–96; 133–141; and 166–172 in *Evidence-based Medicine.*)

[1]You could have found the same reference by doing a MEDLINE literature search on this question, using the search terms 'carotid endarterectomy (as a text word), limited to publication type = randomized-controlled-trial' and the NASCET article would come up. *Best Evidence* was easier and faster for us, and provided both a structured abstract and a commentary from a clinical expert in cerebrovascular disease.

PART

B **How to use the CATMaker (optional)**

If a CATMaker is provided with this package you will be shown how to use it to generate and save your own one page 'critically appraised topic' (CAT) from an article about therapy. The advantages of the CATMaker include its ability to calculate for you the clinically useful measures of the effects of therapy and their confidence intervals, and to save your critical appraisal for printing, sharing and storage.

The New England
Journal of Medicine

©Copyright, 1991, by the Massachusetts Medical Society

| Volume 325 | AUGUST 15, 1991 | Number 7 |

BENEFICIAL EFFECT OF CAROTID ENDARTERECTOMY IN SYMPTOMATIC PATIENTS WITH HIGH-GRADE CAROTID STENOSIS

NORTH AMERICAN SYMPTOMATIC CAROTID ENDARTERECTOMY TRIAL COLLABORATORS*

Abstract *Background.* Without strong evidence of benefit, the use of carotid endarterectomy for prophylaxis against stroke rose dramatically until the mid-1980s, then declined. Our investigation sought to determine whether carotid endarterectomy reduces the risk of stroke among patients with a recent adverse cerebrovascular event and ipsilateral carotid stenosis.

Methods. We conducted a randomized trial at 50 clinical centers throughout the United States and Canada, in patients in two predetermined strata based on the severity of carotid stenosis — 30 to 69 percent and 70 to 99 percent. We report here the results in the 659 patients in the latter stratum, who had had a hemispheric or retinal transient ischemic attack or a nondisabling stroke within the 120 days before entry and had stenosis of 70 to 99 percent in the symptomatic carotid artery. All patients received optimal medical care, including antiplatelet therapy. Those assigned to surgical treatment underwent carotid endarterectomy performed by neurosurgeons or vascular surgeons. All patients were examined by neurologists 1, 3, 6, 9, and 12 months after entry and then every 4 months. End points were assessed by blinded, independent case review. No patient was lost to follow-up.

Results. Life-table estimates of the cumulative risk of any ipsilateral stroke at two years were 26 percent in the 331 medical patients and 9 percent in the 328 surgical patients — an absolute risk reduction (±SE) of 17±3.5 percent (P<0.001). For a major or fatal ipsilateral stroke, the corresponding estimates were 13.1 percent and 2.5 percent — an absolute risk reduction of 10.6±2.6 percent (P<0.001). Carotid endarterectomy was still found to be beneficial when all strokes and deaths were included in the analysis (P<0.001).

Conclusions. Carotid endarterectomy is highly beneficial to patients with recent hemispheric and retinal transient ischemic attacks or nondisabling strokes and ipsilateral high-grade stenosis (70 to 99 percent) of the internal carotid artery. (N Engl J Med 1991; 325:445-53.)

CAROTID endarterectomy was introduced in 1954 as a logical procedure for the prevention of ischemic stroke distal to carotid-artery stenosis.[1] Although the first randomized trials of its effectiveness had negative results,[2-4] surgeons continued to perform carotid endarterectomy and began to report lower rates of perioperative complications.[5,6]

The number of patients undergoing endarterectomy in hospitals in the United States (other than Veterans Affairs hospitals) rose from 15,000 in 1971 to 107,000 in 1985.[7] However, continuing uncertainty about the efficacy of the operation was reflected in marked geographic variation in the rates of endarterectomy.[8] Adding to this uncertainty was the decline in the number of first and fatal strokes,[9-11] the influence of risk-factor management in reducing strokes,[12-14] and emerging recognition of the efficacy of antiplatelet drugs in preventing stroke.[15] When a randomized trial demonstrated that extracranial–intracranial by-pass was ineffective in preventing stroke,[16] this presented an opportunity to reexamine the current efficacy of carotid endarterectomy as performed in North America, and several randomized trials were begun in both symptomatic and asymptomatic patients,[17] complementing the European Carotid Surgery Trial already under way.[18] This report describes the first definitive results of this new round of trials of carotid endarterectomy.

METHODS

A full description of the methods of the study has been published elsewhere.[19] The key features of the conduct of the trial were as follows.

Center Eligibility

The study was conducted at 50 centers in the United States and Canada. Each center had a rate of less than 6 percent for stroke and death occurring within 30 days of operation for at least 50 consecutive carotid endarterectomies performed within the previous 24 months, and each had obtained approval of the research protocol from its local institutional review board.

Patient Eligibility

To be eligible for the trial, patients had to give informed consent, be less than 80 years old, and have had a hemispheric transient ischemic attack (distinct focal neurologic dysfunction) or monocular

*The collaborators in this trial are listed in the Appendix.

Address reprint requests to D.W. Taylor at the Department of Clinical Epidemiology and Biostatistics, McMaster University, 1200 Main St. W., Hamilton, ON L8N 3Z5, Canada, or to Dr. H.J.M. Barnett at the John P. Robarts Research Institute, P.O. Box 5015, 100 Perth Dr., London, ON N6A 5K8, Canada.

Supported by a grant (R01-NS-24456) from the National Institute of Neurological Disorders and Stroke.

blindness persisting less than 24 hours or a nondisabling stroke with persistence of symptoms or signs for more than 24 hours within the previous 120 days, in association with stenosis of 30 to 99 percent in the ipsilateral internal carotid artery; the artery had to be technically suitable for endarterectomy, as assessed by selective carotid angiography.

Using a jeweler's eyepiece marked in tenths of a millimeter, the principal neuroradiologist measured on the angiograms of each patient the luminal diameter (on two views) at the point of greatest stenosis and at the normal part of the artery beyond the carotid bulb. The percent stenosis was determined by calculating the ratio of these two measurements, with use of the view showing the greatest degree of narrowing. If review by the Data Management Center (Robarts Institute) found the stenosis to be less than 30 percent, the angiograms were submitted for independent external adjudication. Patients were categorized at entry as being in one of two predetermined strata: those with 30 to 69 percent stenosis and those with 70 to 99 percent stenosis. The reliability of this assignment was checked in a blinded fashion by the principal neuroradiologist in 127 randomly selected patients; this check revealed a high degree of consistency (kappa = 0.89).

Patients were excluded from the study if they (1) were mentally incompetent or unwilling to give informed consent; (2) had no angiographic visualization of both carotid arteries and their intracranial branches; (3) had an intracranial lesion that was more severe than the surgically accessible lesion; (4) had organ failure of the kidney, liver, or lung, or had cancer judged likely to cause death within five years; (5) had a cerebral infarction on either side that deprived the patient of all useful function in the affected territory; (6) had symptoms that could be attributed to nonatherosclerotic disease (e.g., fibromuscular dysplasia, aneurysm, or tumor); (7) had a cardiac valvular or rhythm disorder likely to be associated with cardioembolic symptoms; or (8) had previously undergone an ipsilateral carotid endarterectomy.

Patients were temporarily ineligible if they had uncontrolled hypertension, diabetes mellitus, or unstable angina pectoris; myocardial infarction within the previous 6 months; signs of progressive neurologic dysfunction; contralateral carotid endarterectomy within the previous 4 months; or a major surgical procedure within the previous 30 days. Such patients could become eligible if the disorder causing their temporary ineligibility resolved within 120 days after their qualifying cerebrovascular event. The data on all ineligible patients and all who were eligible but did not undergo randomization, including all patients undergoing carotid endarterectomy outside the trial, were reported to the Nonrandomized Data Center at the Mayo Clinic.[19]

Base-Line Investigations

Patients underwent standardized history taking, physical and neurologic examinations, a 12-point assessment of functional status, laboratory tests, 12-lead electrocardiography, computerized tomography of the head, angiography and duplex ultrasonography of the carotid arteries, and chest roentgenography.

Randomization

On transmission of base-line data to the Data Management Center, patients were randomly assigned to receive either medical care alone or medical care plus surgery, according to a computer-generated randomization schedule.

Treatment

Antiplatelet treatment (usually 1300 mg of aspirin per day or a lower dose if necessitated by side effects) and, as indicated, antihypertensive, antilipid, and antidiabetic therapy was prescribed for all patients. Those assigned to surgery also underwent carotid endarterectomy. The surgical technique was left to the discretion of the surgeon, and the procedures have been described elsewhere.[19] Simultaneous coronary-artery bypass grafting and simultaneous bilateral carotid endarterectomy were proscribed. Patients with bilateral stenosis who were assigned to surgery could undergo bilateral endarterectomy if the symptomatic side of the carotid was operated on first.

Follow-up

Study surgeons completed postoperative assessments 30 days after surgery or at the time of hospital discharge, whichever occurred first. Study neurologists performed medical, neurologic, and functional-status assessments of all patients one month after entry, then every three months for the first year, and every four months thereafter. The management of cardiovascular risk factors was monitored centrally, and reminders were sent to neurologists if necessary. Computed tomography of the head was performed if cerebrovascular events were suspected. Duplex ultrasonography was repeated one month after entry and after any cerebrovascular event in the carotid distribution. Carotid angiography was repeated after any cerebrovascular event when considered clinically appropriate.

Events

All deaths were assessed for their immediate, underlying, and contributing causes. Strokes were assessed for location, type, laterality, severity, and duration, according to the definitions published by the Committee on Classification of Cerebrovascular Disease of the National Institute of Neurological Disorders and Stroke.[20] New lesions identified on computed tomography were not considered strokes unless appropriate signs or symptoms persisted beyond 24 hours.

Patient eligibility and events were assessed at three levels: by the participating neurologist and surgeon at each center, by the steering committee at the Data Management Center (where a staff neurologist tracked down missing or additional data as needed and then presented each case without revealing treatment assignment), and by a team of blinded external adjudicators who were not otherwise involved in the trial.

Statistical Analysis

The original calculations of sample size allowed for independent analyses in each of four angiographic subgroups defined by the degree of stenosis and angiographic evidence of ulceration. However, the comparison of base-line angiograms and surgical specimens confirmed the insensitivity of angiography in detecting ulceration.[21] Accordingly, this stratification was removed from the primary analyses, leaving just the two strata of high-grade (severe) stenosis (70 to 99 percent) and medium-grade (moderate) stenosis (30 to 69 percent).

All analyses compared medical and surgical patients with respect to the length of time before treatment failure by means of the Mantel–Haenszel chi-square test and Kaplan–Meier survival curves. All reported P values are two-tailed. The primary analysis defined treatment failure as any fatal or nonfatal stroke ipsilateral to the carotid lesion. Other definitions included all strokes and all deaths as well as consideration of the severity of stroke. Strokes producing functional deficits persisting beyond 90 days were considered major. Each of these analyses included all strokes (regardless of location) and all deaths (regardless of cause) that occurred among surgical patients during the 30-day postoperative period and among medical patients during a comparable period after randomization.

Patients found to be ineligible because they did not have either an appropriate carotid lesion or corresponding symptoms were excluded from the primary analysis. Patients who were crossed over to the other treatment group were included in the primary analysis up to the date of crossover, but not after that date.

As dictated in the protocol, monthly interim analyses were initiated in January 1990 (two years after the randomization of the first patient). If the results of any of these monthly analyses, known only to the principal biostatistical investigator and a clinical epidemiologist, showed a difference between the medical and surgical groups that had reached a level of statistical significance of 0.1 percent (P<0.001), the chairman of the National Institutes of Health monitoring committee was to be notified. If this difference remained at the 0.1 percent level over a six-month period, and if the supporting analyses indicated that the interpretation of these results was unambiguous and clinically important, the full monitoring committee was to be convened. The committee was also to be convened if it became possible to rule out, with a high level of confidence, a 10 percent reduction in relative risk as a result of carotid endarterectomy.

Analyses were conducted to ascertain the importance of risk factors by dividing patients into three risk groups of approximately equal size according to a simple count of the commonly recognized risk factors with the use of arbitrary cutoff points: age (>70 years), sex (male), systolic blood pressure (>160 mm Hg), diastolic blood pressure (>90 mm Hg), recency (<31 days) and type of prior cerebrovascular events (stroke, not transient ischemic attack), degree of stenosis (>80 percent), presence of ulceration on the angiogram, and a history of smoking, hypertension, myocardial infarction, congestive heart failure, diabetes, intermittent claudication, or high blood lipid levels. These risk factors and cutoff points were chosen in advance and were not derived through analysis of the data.

RESULTS

Early Termination of the Study in Patients with High-Grade Stenosis

On February 1, 1991, the trial's preplanned rule for stopping randomization was invoked because of evidence of treatment efficacy among patients with high-grade stenosis (70 to 99 percent) who underwent carotid endarterectomy. On February 21, the monitoring and executive committees agreed that (1) randomization of patients with high-grade stenosis should be stopped, (2) a summary of the results in the patients with high-grade stenosis should be communicated immediately to the participating clinicians, along with a list of all patients given medical treatment alone to whom the results might apply, (3) reports of all strokes and deaths and all patient assessments occurring before February 21 should be collected as quickly as possible for inclusion in this report, and (4) the parallel study dealing with symptomatic patients with medium-grade stenosis (30 to 69 percent) should be continued. The sponsoring agency, the National Institute of Neurological Disorders and Stroke, independently issued a peer-reviewed Clinical Alert to convey immediately a summary of these interim results to physicians across North America.

Patient Entry

Six hundred sixty-two patients with high-grade carotid stenosis (determined by central radiologic review) were enrolled between January 1, 1988, and February 21, 1991. Of these, three patients (0.5 percent) were subsequently excluded from the primary analysis by a blinded review panel because they did not meet entry criteria: one (assigned to surgical treatment) had symptoms due solely to glaucoma, one (assigned to medical therapy) had symptoms of a vertebrobasilar transient ischemic attack only, and one (assigned to surgical treatment) had occlusion of the internal carotid artery. Randomization created balanced treatment groups with respect to the qualifying cerebrovascular events, underlying vascular lesions, and important prognostic characteristics (Table 1).

Table 1. Base-Line Characteristics of the Treatment Groups.

CHARACTERISTIC	MEDICAL (N = 331)	SURGICAL (N = 328)
Median age (yr)	66	65
	% of group	
Sex		
Male	69	68
Female	31	32
Transient ischemic attack at entry	69	67
Stroke at entry	31	33
Ipsilateral stenosis		
70–79%	43	40
80–89%	33	38
90–99%	24	22
Contralateral stenosis, 70–99%	9	8
Race		
White	89	93
Black	4	2
Other	7	5
Prior myocardial infarction	18	18
Stable angina pectoris	25	22
Hypertension	61	60
Diabetes	21	17
Hyperlipidemia	25	21
Intermittent claudication	16	15
Current cigarette smoking	33	37
Antithrombotic medications	85	85

The similarity between the patients included and those excluded, reported elsewhere,[19] confirmed that no subgroup of eligible patients was systematically excluded from the trial.

Patient Follow-up

No patient was lost to follow-up and none withdrew; 98 percent of the surviving patients had their last follow-up examination within 4 months of the February 21 closing date, and the average duration of follow-up was 18 months. Twenty-one medical patients (6.3 percent) were crossed over and underwent carotid endarterectomy on the same side as the lesion for which they were randomized (10 after transient ischemic attacks, 6 after a stroke, 2 as a prelude to other required surgery, 2 after refusing the random assignment, and 1 on the advice of a nonparticipating physician). Of the 328 patients assigned to surgery, only 1 refused the operation and received medical treatment alone. All the others underwent carotid endarterectomy, performed an average of two days after randomization. Medical regimens to reduce the risk of stroke were applied equally in both treatment groups. At the last reported follow-up examination, antihypertensive therapy was being given to 187 medical patients (57 percent) and 178 surgical patients (54 percent); elevation of the diastolic blood pressure (>95 mm Hg) was significantly more prevalent among the surgical patients than the medical patients (13 percent vs. 8 percent, P<0.05). Over 99 percent of both medical and surgical patients were taking antithrombotic drugs at the last follow-up visit, most commonly aspirin, which was being used by 94 percent of the medical patients and 98 percent of the surgical patients.

Perioperative Morbidity and Mortality

The perioperative period was considered the time from randomization to 30 days after surgery (which was performed a median of 2 days after randomization). None of the 328 surgical patients had a stroke or died between randomization and surgery. In the perioperative period, 18 surgical patients (5.5 percent) had cerebrovascular events; 12 events were minor, 5 were major (i.e., causing a functional deficit persisting ≥90 days), and 1 was fatal. In addition, one patient died suddenly after surgery, for a rate of 5.8 percent for all perioperative stroke and death. Restricting the analysis to the most serious events resulted in a rate of 2.1 percent for major stroke and death and a fatality rate of 0.6 percent.

In the comparable 32-day period after randomization among the 331 medical patients, 11 (3.3 percent) had cerebrovascular events; 8 events were minor, 2 were major, and 1 was fatal. This resulted in a rate of 3.3 percent for all stroke and death within 32 days of randomization, which included a rate of 0.9 percent for major stroke and death and a fatality rate of 0.3 percent.

Other surgical complications included cranial-nerve injury (7.6 percent), wound hematoma (5.5 percent), wound infection (3.4 percent), myocardial infarction (0.9 percent), congestive heart failure (0.6 percent), arrhythmia (1.2 percent), and other cardiovascular problems (1.2 percent). Of these complications, 81 percent were considered mild (of no lasting consequence and not prolonging hospitalization) and the rest were considered moderate (of no lasting consequence but prolonging the hospital stay).

Events

As shown in the first row of Table 2, the life-table estimate of the risk of any fatal or nonfatal ipsilateral stroke by 24 months after randomization was 26 percent for the medical patients and only 9 percent for the surgical patients (including any stroke or death occurring postoperatively or within 32 days of randomization), resulting in an absolute risk reduction of 17 percent. Thus, for every 100 patients treated surgically, 17 were spared an ipsilateral stroke over the next two years. This represents a relative-risk reduction of 65 percent and shows that six such patients are the "number needed to be treated"[22] in order to prevent one adverse event by 24 months. The second through sixth rows of Table 2 show that carotid endarterectomy remained beneficial with respect to each of the five other definitions of outcome events.

The vast majority of first events were ipsilateral strokes (61 in medical patients vs. 26 in surgical patients), and although the overall difference between the treatment groups remained significant when other

Table 2. First Adverse Events and Actuarial Failure Rates at Two Years of Follow-up, According to the Event Defining Treatment Failure.

Event Defining Failure*	Medical Patients (N = 331)	Surgical Patients (N = 328)	Absolute Difference ±SE	Relative-Risk Reduction
	events (event rate, %†)		%	%
Any ipsilateral stroke	61 (26.0)	26 (9.0)	17.0±3.5‡	65
Any stroke	64 (27.6)	34 (12.6)	15.0±3.8‡	54
Any stroke or death	73 (32.3)	41 (15.8)	16.5±4.2‡	51
Major or fatal ipsilateral stroke	29 (13.1)	8 (2.5)	10.6±2.6‡	81
Any major or fatal stroke	29 (13.1)	10 (3.7)	9.4±2.7‡	72
Any major stroke or death	38 (18.1)	19 (8.0)	10.1±3.5§	56

*"Death" refers to mortality from all causes. In addition to the events defining treatment failure, each value includes all strokes (any severity and any site) and deaths from any cause: in the surgical patients, between randomization and the 30th day after surgery, and in the medical patients, during the comparable 32-day period beginning with randomization.

†Failure rates were derived from Kaplan–Meier estimates of survival.

‡P<0.001 for the comparison of the treatment groups.

§P<0.01 for the comparison of the treatment groups.

events were included, carotid endarterectomy proved beneficial in that it reduced ipsilateral strokes. The inclusion of stroke in the distribution of the contralateral carotid and vertebral basilar arteries added only three events to those in the medical group and eight to those in the surgical group, and the further addition of death from any cause added another nine and seven events, respectively. The treatment groups did not differ significantly in total mortality (Table 3).

Survival curves for the values reflected in each of the rows in Table 2 are shown in Figure 1. They reveal two additional points of interest. First, the early disadvantage to the surgical patients (who faced a risk of perioperative stroke and death) was rapidly overcome, with the curves for the medical and the surgical patients crossing about three months after randomization. Second, there was no evidence of convergence of the two curves for as long as 30 months, indicating that the beneficial effects of surgery persisted at least this long.

Among the patients who did not die or have a major stroke during the first month after randomization, the

Table 3. Total Mortality According to Treatment Group.

Cause of Death	Medical (N = 331)	Surgical (N = 328)
	no. of patients	
Stroke	5	2
Myocardial infarction	4	4
Other ischemic heart disease	3	1
Sudden death	1	3
Other cardiovascular disease	1	0
Cancer	2	2
Respiratory disease	1	1
Other cause	4	2
Total — no. (%)	21 (6.3)	15 (4.6)

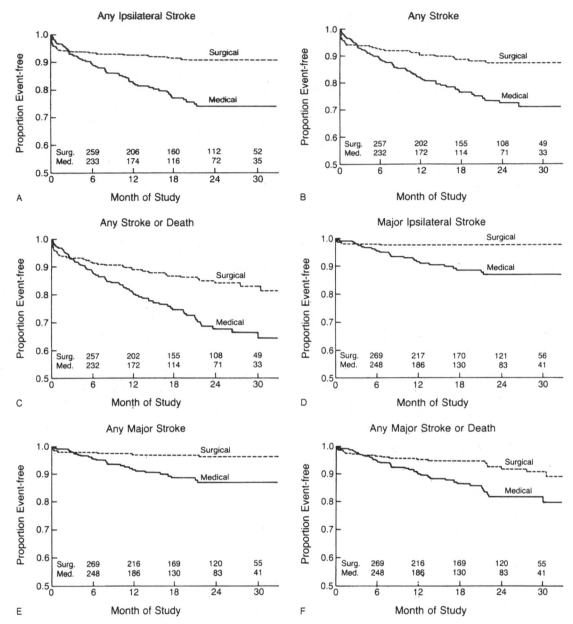

Figure 1. Survival Curves for the Treatment Groups.

These Kaplan–Meier survival curves show the probability of surviving six events indicating treatment failure after randomization. The number of patients who remained event-free in each treatment group is shown at six-month intervals at the bottom of each graph; the numbers at time zero are 328 in the surgical group and 331 in the medical group. The curves of the groups differed significantly (by Mantel–Haenszel chi-square test, P<0.001 for all events except "any major stroke or death," for which P<0.01).

risk of any major or fatal stroke within two years was 12.2 percent in the medical group and 1.6 percent in the surgical group (P<0.00001). Thus, the immediate postoperative increase in the risk of major stroke or death among the surgical patients, 1.2 percent (2.1 percent − 0.9 percent), was offset by an absolute

risk reduction of 10.6 percent for major or fatal stroke during the subsequent two years.

Analyzing our results according to the intention-to-treat principle produced essentially the same levels of significance and standard errors for between-group differences. This analysis, which included the three

Session 1 – Therapy & introduction to CATs

incorrectly randomized ineligible patients and counted events occurring in a patient after crossover according to the group to which the patient had originally been assigned, added just one event to those in the medical group and two events to those in the surgical group. The analyses reported in this paper include 30 patients found to be technically ineligible because of inadequate angiography (17 patients), severe intracranial stenosis (4), cerebral aneurysms (3), cardiac disorders (3), and other medical problems (3). Excluding these patients from the analysis reduced by five the events in the medical group and by three the events in the surgical group and did not alter the interpretation of the results. An analysis comparing results at large centers with those at small centers, and results at U.S. centers with those at Canadian centers, revealed no significant differences in the benefit of surgery according to the size or country of a study center.

The proportion of medical patients who had an ipsilateral stroke within two years was 17 percent in the low-risk group (0 to 5 risk factors), 23 percent in the moderate-risk group (6 risk factors), and 39 percent in the high-risk group ($\geq$7 risk factors) ($P<0.001$). The prognosis of the surgical patients did not vary significantly among risk groups and averaged 9 percent at two years.

A secondary analysis showed that finer divisions of the degree of high-grade carotid stenosis (i.e., 70 to 79, 80 to 89, and 90 to 99 percent) correlated with the degrees of risk reduction after surgery. The absolute risk reduction ($\pm$SE) for all ipsilateral stroke at two years was 26$\pm$8.1 percent among patients with stenosis of 90 to 99 percent at entry, 18$\pm$6.2 percent among those with stenosis of 80 to 89 percent, and 12$\pm$4.8 percent among those with stenosis of 70 to 79 percent.

DISCUSSION

Among symptomatic patients with high-grade stenosis (70 to 99 percent), those who underwent carotid endarterectomy had an absolute reduction of 17 percent in the risk of ipsilateral stroke at two years ($P<0.001$). This benefit was not diminished when strokes in other carotid and vertebral basilar territories and deaths from all causes were included in the analysis. Furthermore, clinically important and statistically significant beneficial effects persisted when the analyses excluded minor and nondisabling strokes and when they included patients with protocol violations.

Similar results have recently been reported from the European Carotid Surgery Trial.[18] Among 778 symptomatic patients with severe stenosis (70 to 99 percent) who were randomly assigned to treatment with carotid endarterectomy or medical care alone, 7.5 percent of the surgical patients had an ipsilateral stroke or died within 30 days of surgery. Life-table estimates of the risk of ipsilateral stroke during the next three years yielded an additional risk of 2.8 percent for surgical

patients, as compared with 16.8 percent for medical patients ($P<0.0001$). The European study also concluded that the immediate risks of surgery outweighed any potential long-term benefit in the 374 symptomatic patients with mild stenosis (0 to 29 percent). Because definitive conclusions are not yet possible, both the European and North American trials are being continued in patients with moderate stenosis (30 to 69 percent).

After surgery, we observed no significant difference in event rates among patients with different numbers of base-line risk factors. Thus, the degree of benefit that individual patients received from carotid endarterectomy was directly proportional to the risk they faced without surgery, and those with the highest risk at entry gained the most. Our original estimates of the risk of stroke (4 to 7 percent per year), based on results in placebo groups in trials of antithrombotic drugs, substantially underestimated the risk of stroke among symptomatic patients with high-grade stenosis. The life-table estimates of the risk of stroke at two years among our medical patients were 26 percent for ipsilateral stroke, 28 percent for stroke in any territory, and 32 percent for any stroke or death.

We caution readers not to apply our conclusions too broadly. First, the study surgeons were selected only after audits of their endarterectomy results by our surgical committee confirmed a high level of expertise. If comparable expertise and quality control are not achieved in the widespread implementation of these results and the perioperative risk of major stroke and death exceeds the 2.1 percent reported here, the benefit of endarterectomy will diminish. If the rate of major complications approaches 10 percent, the benefit will vanish entirely. Second, our method of measuring stenosis was strict. The results reported here relate only to patients in whom the ratio of the narrowest diameter of the diseased artery (the numerator) to the diameter of the artery beyond the bulb and beyond recognizable disease involvement (the denominator) indicated stenosis of 70 to 99 percent. Our results do not apply if the diameter of the carotid bulb or a segment with poststenotic dilatation is used as the denominator of this ratio in the measurement of stenosis (the severity of stenosis would be overestimated). Third, we have no information about the efficacy of endarterectomy in patients whose ischemic events occur more than 120 days before surgery or who either have already had a devastating stroke or are in the throes of a progressing stroke. Nor did our study include patients who had failure of other major organs or heart disorders that might produce emboli. Also, as indicated by the preponderance of ipsilateral stroke, the patients included in this study did not have widespread cerebrovascular disease.

Patients in both treatment groups underwent cervical and intracranial carotid arteriography before randomization in order to rule out the presence of distal disease more severe than that in the surgically accessible cervical carotid artery. Because a major stroke complicating arteriography would preclude admission to the trial, the benefits reported here should be adjusted downward to include the risk of arteriography. The risk of major stroke or death due to angiography should be no more than 1 percent in patients studied because of arteriosclerotic disease of the cerebral arteries.[23-25] If the decision to perform angiography were based on the results of noninvasive ultrasound examination, patients with lesser degrees of stenosis could be spared the risks of angiography. A rigorous comparison of ultrasound with angiography in symptomatic patients would be required to give a precise estimate of the effect of this diagnostic strategy.

In our group of patients with high-grade stenosis, those with less severe stenosis had a lower risk of stroke, and their gains from surgery were smaller than those of patients with more severe stenosis. This observation reinforces a continuing uncertainty about the efficacy of carotid endarterectomy for stenosis in the range of 30 to 69 percent. The investigators in both the North American and the European trials are continuing to study symptomatic patients with moderate stenosis (30 to 69 percent). Together these trials will determine whether patients with this degree of stenosis will benefit from endarterectomy, and if so, will identify the point at which the risks of surgery outweigh its benefits.

The effects of publishing the results of both trials on the future frequency of carotid endarterectomy will be followed with considerable interest. Over the past few years, many referring physicians have shown a declining interest in carotid endarterectomy and have acted as if the absence of proof were the proof of absence. In 1985, 107,000 carotid endarterectomies were performed in hospitals (excluding Veterans Affairs hospitals) in the United States. By 1989, the number had diminished to 70,000 (Dyken ML, Pokras R: personal communication). In the light of the results reported here, this reduction in the number of carotid endarterectomies may have deprived some patients with high-grade stenosis of what is now confirmed to be a beneficial operation.

On the basis of these results and those of the European trial, patients with transient ischemic attacks or recent minor strokes without an obvious cardiac cause, who are otherwise fit for surgery, should be screened with noninvasive ultrasonographic techniques. Those with minimal narrowing or none should be treated with what is currently the best medical care. Those with moderate or severe narrowing should be seriously considered for arteriography. If those shown by arteriography to have moderate stenosis (30 to 69 percent) are referred to one of the study centers of the North American trial, the part of the trial focusing on moderate stenosis will be concluded sooner. Patients with high-grade stenosis (70 to 99 percent) should be considered for referral to institutions and surgeons who practice vigorous quality control and have the low rates of perioperative morbidity and mortality that have characterized the centers and physicians in this trial.

These positive findings among symptomatic patients with high-grade stenosis provide no answers to the question of the optimal treatment of patients with asymptomatic carotid stenosis. It is essential that the trials under way to study such patients be continued.

Appendix

The following persons and institutions participated in the North American Symptomatic Carotid Endarterectomy Trial:

Steering and Writing Committee of the Executive Committee: Principal Investigator — Henry J.M. Barnett, M.D. (John P. Robarts Research Institute); Co-Principal Investigators — D.W. Taylor, M.A. (biostatistics; Chairman, Writing Committee), R.B. Haynes, M.D. (epidemiology), and D.L. Sackett, M.D. (epidemiology) (McMaster University); S.J. Peerless, M.D. (surgery), G.G. Ferguson, M.D. (surgery), A.J. Fox, M.D. (neuroradiology), R.N. Rankin, M.D. (neurosonography), and V.C. Hachinski, M.D. (neurology) (University of Western Ontario); D.O. Wiebers, M.D. (neurology) (Mayo Clinic); and M. Eliasziw, Ph.D. (biostatistics) (John P. Robarts Research Institute). *Additional Members of Executive Committee (current and past):* H.W.K. Barr, M.D., G.P. Clagett, M.D., J.D. Easton, M.D., J.W. Harbison, M.D., R.C. Heros, M.D., A.R. Hudson, M.D., J.R. Marler, M.D., R.A. Ratcheson, M.D., D. Sim, Ph.D., D. Simard, M.D., M.D. Walker, M.D., P.M. Walker, M.D., and P.A. Wolf, M.D. *Surgical Committee:* S.J. Peerless, M.D. (Chairman), G.G. Ferguson, M.D. (Secretary), G.P. Clagett, M.D., R.C. Heros, M.D., A.R. Hudson, M.D., R.H. Patterson, M.D., M. Webster, M.D., R.A. Ratcheson, M.D., and P.M. Walker, M.D.

The participating centers, in order of the number of eligible patients entered, were as follows: *University of Western Ontario (University Hospital and St. Joseph's Health Centre), London, Ont.:* V.C. Hachinski, M.D. (Principal Investigator), C. Swan, R.N. (Coordinator), C. White, R.N. (Coordinator), G.G. Ferguson, M.D., S.J. Peerless, M.D., and H. Reichman, M.D.; *University of Toronto, Toronto:* F.L. Silver, M.D. (Principal Investigator), B. Huth (Coordinator), S. Slattery (Coordinator), N.H. Bayer, M.D., D.S. Borrett, M.D., V.M. Campbell, M.D., J.F.R. Fleming, M.D., F. Gentili, M.D., M.A. Keller, M.D., R.J. Moulton, M.D., P.J. Muller, M.D., P.M. Walker, M.D., and M.C. Wallace, M.D.; *Virginia Commonwealth University, Richmond:* J.W. Harbison, M.D. (Principal Investigator), P. Rosenfeld, R.N. (Coordinator), W.L. Felton III, M.D., H.M. Lee, M.D., J.P. Muizelaar, M.D., M. Sobel, M.D., W. Stringer, M.D., and J.R. Taylor, M.D.; *University of British Columbia, Vancouver:* V.P. Sweeney, M.D. (Principal Investigator), J.L. Bloomer, R.N. (Coordinator), D. Cameron, M.D., R. Nugent, M.D., J. Reid, M.D., A.J. Salvian, M.D., J.G. Sladen, M.D., and P. Teal, M.D.; *University of Western Ontario (Victoria Hospital), London, Ont.:* J.D. Spence, M.D. (Principal Investigator), L. Sykes, R.N. (Coordinator), B. Tate, R.N. (Coordinator), H.W.K. Barr, M.D., K. Harris, M.D., and W. Pexman, M.D.; *Laval University (Hôpital de l'Enfant-Jesus), Quebec City, Que.:* D. Simard, M.D. (Principal Investigator), A. Lajeunesse, R.N. (Coordinator), J.M. Bouchard, M.D., J. Cote, M.D., D. Marois, M.D., C. Roberge, M.D., and J.F. Turcotte, M.D.; *University of Ottawa, Ottawa, Ont.:* B.G. Benoit, M.D. (Principal Investigator), I. Polis (Coordinator), T. Polis, M.D. (Coordinator), E.A. Atack, M.D., D.M. Atack, M.D., A. Buchan, M.D., J.M.E.G. Belanger, M.D., G.H. Embree, M.D., D.N. Preston, M.D., and N. Russell, M.D.; *University of Oregon, Portland:* B.M. Coull, M.D. (Principal Investigator), P. de Garmo, A.N.P. (Coordinator), P. Marshall (Coordinator), D. Briley, M.D., G. Moneta, M.D., S. Roman-Goldstein, M.D., and R. Yeager, M.D.; *Marshfield Medical Research Foundation, Marshfield, Wis.:* P. Karanjia, M.D. (Principal Investigator), C. Matti, R.N. (Coordinator), L. O'Rourke (Coordinator), B. Brink, M.D., R. Carlson, M.D.,

B. Hiner, M.D., L. Kolts, M.D., M. Kuehner, M.D., K. Madden, M.D., and M. Swanson, M.D.; *University of Montreal, Montreal:* L.H. Lebrun, M.D. (Principal Investigator), M.P. Desrochers, R.N. (Coordinator), A. Bellavance, M.D., L. Choimiere, M.D., P. Couillard, M.D., N. Daneault, M.D., M. Duplessis, M.D., S. Fontaine, M.D., S. Lauzier, M.D., J. Raymond, M.D., G. Rowny, M.D., and A. Sfier, M.D.; *University of Iowa, Iowa City:* H. Adams, M.D. (Principal Investigator), V. Mitchell, R.N. (Coordinator), J. Biller, M.D., S.H. Cornell, M.D., J.D. Corson, M.D., and C. Loftus, M.D.; *Dartmouth College, Hanover, N.H.:* A.G. Reeves, M.D. (Principal Investigator), P. Orem, B.S., R.N. (Coordinator), L. Cromwell, M.D., R.E. Harbaugh, M.D., and R.E. Nordgren, M.D.; *Laval University (Hôpital St.-Sacrement), Quebec City, Que.:* E. Daigle, M.D. (Principal Investigator), L. Lessard, R.N. (Coordinator), Y. Douville, M.D., R. Labbe, M.D., F. Laroche, M.D., and H.P. Noel, M.D.; *McGill University (Montreal General Hospital), Montreal:* R. Cote, M.D. (Principal Investigator), F. Bourque, R.N. (Coordinator), S. Campion, R.N. (Coordinator), J.L. Caron, M.D., J.D. Chan, M.D., R. Ford, M.D., and D.S. Mulder, M.D.; *Sunnybrook Medical Center, Toronto:* J.W. Norris, M.D. (Principal Investigator), B. Bowyer (Coordinator), J. Twiner (Coordinator), P.W. Cooper, M.D., M. Fazl, M.D., M.J. Gawel, M.D., R. Maggisano, M.D., and D.W. Rowed, M.D.; *University of Texas, Dallas:* G.P. Clagett, M.D. (Principal Investigator), J.A. Heller, R.N. (Coordinator), A. Pruitt, R.N. (Coordinator), S. Myers, M.D., P. Purdy, M.D., and H. Unwin, M.D.; *Mississauga Hospital, Mississauga, Ont.:* G. Sawa, M.D. (Principal Investigator), G. Barnard (Coordinator), C. Kennedy, R.N. (Coordinator), V. Ozolins, M.D., and H. Schutz, M.D.; *University of Minnesota, Minneapolis:* S. Haines, M.D. (Principal Investigator), N. Olson, R.N. (Coordinator), J. Abel, R.N. (Coordinator), J. Davenport, M.D., R.C. Heros, M.D., M.J. Nelson, M.D., and D.A. Turner, M.D.; *University of Pittsburgh, Pittsburgh:* O. Reinmuth, M.D. (Principal Investigator), S. DeCesare (Coordinator), M. Webster, M.D., and L. Wechsler, M.D.; *University of Manitoba, Winnipeg:* B. Anderson, M.D. (Principal Investigator), D. Gladish, R.N. (Coordinator), A. Auty, M.D., B. McClarty, M.D., G. Sutherland, M.D., and M. West, M.D.; *Brown University, Providence, R.I.:* J.D. Easton, M.D. (Principal Investigator), J.A. Sarafin, R.N. (Coordinator), R.A. Haas, M.D., and N. Knuckey, M.D.; *State University of New York, Syracuse:* A. Culebras, M.D. (Principal Investigator), J. Drucker, R.N. (Coordinator), C. Law, R.N. (Coordinator), E. Cacayorin, M.D., and C. Hodge, M.D.; *McMaster University, Hamilton, Ont.:* R. Duke, M.D. (Principal Investigator), P. Trevisani, R.N. (Coordinator), M. Alesi, R.N. (Coordinator), M. Molot, M.D., and J.D. Wells, M.D.; *Ohio State University, Columbus:* A.P. Slivka, M.D. (Principal Investigator), T. Brink, R.N. (Coordinator), J. Durham, M.D., W.L. Smead, M.D., A.E. Stockum, M.D., and J.G. Wright, M.D.; *University of Texas, San Antonio:* D.G. Sherman, M.D. (Principal Investigator), C. Sherman, R.N. (Coordinator), C. Easton, R.N. (Coordinator), R.G. Hart, M.D., W. Rogers, M.D., H.D. Root, M.D., and C. Tegeler, M.D.; *University of Calgary, Calgary, Alb.:* K.M. Hoyte, M.D. (Principal Investigator), M. Robertson, R.N. (Coordinator), K.M. Hunter, M.D., S.T. Myles, M.D., R. Ramsay, M.D., H.A. Swanson, M.D., and B.I. Tranmer, M.D.; *University of Missouri, Columbia:* J. Byer, M.D. (Principal Investigator), C. Kelley, R.N. (Coordinator), M.K. Gumerlock, M.D., M. Nelson, M.D., and J. Oro, M.D.; *University of Southern California, Los Angeles:* M. Fisher, M.D. (Principal Investigator), J. Ahmadi, M.D., S. Ameriso, M.D. (Coordinator), F. Weaver, M.D., and A.E. Yellin, M.D.; *Dalhousie University, Halifax, N.S.:* C.W. McCormick, M.D. (Principal Investigator), J. McCormick, R.N. (Coordinator), R.O. Holness, M.D., W.J. Howes, M.D., G. Llewellyn, M.D., D. Malloy, M.D., and S. Phillips, M.D.; *University of Miami, Miami:* R.E. Kelley, Jr., M.D. (Principal Investigator), L. Solari, R.N., B.S.N. (Coordinator), R. Safon, R.N. (Coordinator), J. Kochan, M.D., and A.S. Livingstone, M.D.; *University of Texas, Houston:* J. Grotta, M.D. (Principal Investigator), P. Bratina, R.N. (Coordinator), G. Clifton, M.D., and J. Yeakley, M.D.; *Albert Einstein College of Medicine, Bronx, N.Y.:* D. Rosenbaum, M.D. (Principal Investigator), E. Klonowski, R.N. (Coordinator), R. de los Reyes, M.D., S. Gupta, M.D., F. Moser, M.D., F. Veith, M.D., and K. Wengerter, M.D.; *Boston University, Boston:* P.A. Wolf, M.D. (Principal Investigator), E. Licata-Gehr, R.N., M.S.N. (Coordinator), N.C. Allen, R.N., M.S.N. (Coordinator), V.L. Babikian, M.D., N. Cantelmo, M.D., C.S. Kase, M.D., and J.O. Menzoian, M.D.; *St. Louis University, St. Louis:* C. Gomez, M.D. (Principal Investigator), M. Jedlicka, R.N. (Coordinator), Y. Yusufaly, M.D. (Coordinator), E. Awwad, M.D., R. Bucholz, M.D., and K.R. Smith, Jr., M.D.; *University of Alberta, Edmonton:* M.G. Elleker, M.D. (Principal Investigator), E. Hutchings, R.N. (Coordinator), G. Andrew, M.D., R. Ashforth, M.D., B. Bharadwaj, M.D., and J.M. Findlay, M.D.; *University of Illinois, Chicago/Peoria:* C.M. Helgason, M.D. (Principal Investigator), S. Clemons, R.N. (Coordinator), J. Arzbaecher, R.N. (Coordinator), M. Budi, R.N. (Coordinator), R. Crowell, M.D., J. DeBord, M.D., and J. Schuler, M.D.; *University of Mississippi, Jackson:* R.R. Smith, M.D. (Principal Investigator), R.L. Brown, R.N. (Coordinator), A.F. Haerer, M.D., and W. Russell, M.D.; *Beth Israel Hospital, Boston:* C. Mayman, M.D. (Principal Investigator), M. Tijerina, R.N. (Coordinator), K.C. Kent, M.D., J. Kleefield, M.D., and J.J. Skillman, M.D.; *Temple University, Philadelphia:* R.H. Rosenwasser, M.D. (Principal Investigator), G. Larese-Ortiz (Coordinator), B. Tournier (Coordinator), A.J. Comerota, M.D., D. Jamieson, M.D., and T. Liu, M.D.; *McGill University (Jewish General Hospital/Notre Dame Hospital), Montreal:* G. Mohr, M.D. (Principal Investigator), S. Entis, R.N. (Coordinator), P. LaPlante, R.N. (Coordinator), S. Brem, M.D., J. Carlton, M.D., and M. Goldenberg, M.D.; *University of Tennessee, Memphis:* J.T. Robertson, M.D. (Principal Investigator), J. Riley, R.N. (Coordinator), J. Connell, R.N. (Coordinator), F. Eggers, M.D., and S. Erkulwater, M.D.; *Barrow Neurological Institute, Phoenix, Ariz.:* R. Spetzler, M.D. (Principal Investigator), H. Jahnke, R.N. (Coordinator), J. Frey, M.D., and J. Hodak, M.D.; *University of Saskatchewan, Saskatoon:* A. Shuaib, M.D. (Principal Investigator), C. Regier, R.N. (Coordinator), and F.M. Denath, M.D.; *Memorial University, St. John's, Newf.:* A.E. Goodridge, M.D. (Principal Investigator), K. Murphy, R.N. (Coordinator), A. Badejo, M.D., and M. Mangan, M.D.; *Good Samaritan Hospital, Cincinnati:* R.E. Welling, M.D. (Principal Investigator), D. Feldman, B.A. (Coordinator), R. Lukin, M.D., and R.L. Reed, M.D.; *University of California, San Diego:* J. Rothrock, M.D. (Principal Investigator), N. Kelly, R.N. (Coordinator), K. Hogan, R.N. (Coordinator), R.J. Hye, M.D., and J. Hesselink, M.D.; *University of New Mexico, Albuquerque:* L. Kesterson, M.D. (Principal Investigator), L. Rivera, R.N. (Coordinator), K. Martinez, R.N. (Coordinator), A. Bruno, M.D., and A. Champlin, M.D.; *Wadsworth Veterans Affairs Hospital, Los Angeles:* S.N. Cohen, M.D. (Principal Investigator), J. Kawafuchi, R.N. (Coordinator), J.G. Frazee, M.D., J. Freischlag, M.D., N. Martin, M.D., G. Peters, M.D., and G. White, M.D.; *Neurological Institute, New York:* J.P. Mohr, M.D. (Principal Investigator), A. Cruz, R.N. (Coordinator), S.K. Hilal, M.D., and D. Quest, M.D.

Management Staff (Mayo Clinic, McMaster University, and the John P. Robarts Research Institute): L. Bailey, P. Beattie, B. Bergman, E. Bosch, R. Cook, M. Douglas, J. French, M.J. Gagnon, M.J. Livingstone, H. Meldrum, D. Pahl, D. Kaderabek, J. Richardson, B. Sharpe, C. Swan, C. White, and M. Wright; Staff Neurologists — O. Benavente, M.D., M. Brown, M.D., I. Meissner, M.D., T. Mirsen, M.D., and J. Streifler, M.D. *Adjudicating Committee:* T. Brott, M.D. (neurologist), J. D'Alton, M.D. (neurologist), R. Gunton, M.D. (cardiologist), I. Kricheff, M.D. (neuroradiologist), J. Little, M.D. (neurosurgeon), T. Riles, M.D. (vascular surgeon), J. Robertson, M.D. (neurosurgeon), and G. Wortzman, M.D. (neuroradiologist). *Monitoring Committee:* M.D. Walker, M.D. (Chairman, National Institute of Neurological Disorders and Stroke), B. Brown, Jr., Ph.D. (Stanford University), E.S. Flamm, M.D. (New York University), A.M. Imparato, M.D. (New York University), J.R. Marler, M.D. (National Institute of Neurological Disorders and Stroke), R.G. Ojemann, M.D. (Massachusetts General Hospital), W. Powers, M.D. (Washington University), T. Price, M.D. (University of Maryland), and D.E. Strandness, M.D. (University of Washington).

REFERENCES

1. Eastcott HHG, Pickering GW, Rob CG. Reconstruction of internal carotid artery in a patient with intermittent attacks of hemiplegia. Lancet 1954; 2:994-6.
2. Fields WS, Maslenikov V, Meyer JS, Hass WK, Remington RD, Macdonald M. Joint study of extracranial arterial occlusion. V. Progress report of prognosis following surgery or nonsurgical treatment for transient cerebral ischemic attacks and cervical carotid artery lesions. JAMA 1970; 211:1993-2003.
3. Kurtzke J. Formal discussion. In: Whisnant JP, Sandok BA, eds. Cerebral vascular disease–Ninth Princeton Conference. New York: Grune & Stratton, 1974:190-3.
4. Shaw DA, Venables GS, Cartlidge NEF, Bates D, Dickinson PH. Carotid endarterectomy in patients with transient cerebral ischaemia. J Neurol Sci 1984; 64:45-53.
5. Baker WH, Littooy FN, Greisler HP. et al. Carotid endarterectomy in private practice by fellowship-trained surgeons. Stroke 1987; 5:957-8.
6. Sundt TM Jr, Whisnant JP, Houser OW, Fode NC. Prospective study of the effectiveness and durability of carotid endarterectomy. Mayo Clin Proc 1990; 65:625-35.
7. Pokras R, Dyken ML. Dramatic changes in the performance of endarterectomy for diseases of the extracranial arteries of the head. Stroke 1988; 19:1289-90.
8. Warlow CP. Carotid endarterectomy: does it work? Stroke 1984; 15:1068-76.
9. Bonita R, Stewart A, Beaglehole R. International trends in stroke mortality: 1970–1985. Stroke 1990; 21:989-92.
10. Kotila M. Decline in the incidence of stroke. Stroke 1988; 19:1572-3.
11. Arraiz GA. Mortality patterns from 1931 to 1986 of Canadians aged 35 to 64. Chronic Dis Can 1989; 10:22-7.
12. Shinton R, Beevers G. Meta-analysis of relation between cigarette smoking and stroke. BMJ 1989; 298:789-94.
13. Klag MJ, Whelton PK, Seidler AJ. Decline in US stroke mortality: demographic trends and antihypertensive treatment. Stroke 1989; 20:14-21.
14. Garraway WM, Whisnant JP. The changing pattern of hypertension and the declining incidence of stroke. JAMA 1987; 258:214-7.
15. Antiplatelet Trialists' Collaboration. Secondary prevention of vascular disease by prolonged antiplatelet treatment. BMJ 1988; 296:320-31.
16. The EC/IC Bypass Study Group. Failure of extracranial–intracranial arterial bypass to reduce the risk of ischemic stroke: results of an international randomized trial. N Engl J Med 1985; 313:1191-200.
17. Barnett HJM. Symptomatic carotid endarterectomy trials. Stroke 1990; 21:Suppl 11:III-2–III-5.
18. European Carotid Surgery Trialists' Collaborative Group. MRC European Carotid Surgery Trial: interim results for symptomatic patients with severe (70-99%) or with mild (0-29%) carotid stenosis. Lancet 1991; 337:1235-43.
19. North American Symptomatic Carotid Endarterectomy Trial (NASCET) Steering Committee. North American Symptomatic Carotid Endarterectomy Trial: methods, patient characteristics, and progress. Stroke 1991; 22:711-20.
20. Special report from the National Institute of Neurological Disorders and Stroke. Classification of cerebrovascular diseases III. Stroke 1990; 21:637-76.
21. Streifler JY, Benavente OR, Fox AJ. The accuracy of angiographic detection of carotid plaque ulceration: results from the NASCET study. Stroke 1991; 22:149. abstract.
22. Laupacis A, Sackett DL, Roberts RS. An assessment of clinically useful measures of the consequences of treatment. N Engl J Med 1988; 318:1728-33.
23. Dion JE, Gates PC, Fox AJ, Barnett HJM, Blom RJ. Clinical events following neuroangiography: a prospective study. Stroke 1987; 18:997-1004.
24. Hankey GJ, Warlow CP, Sellar RJ. Cerebral angiographic risk in mild cerebrovascular disease. Stroke 1990; 21:209-22.
25. Earnest F IV, Forbes G, Sandok BA, et al. Complications of cerebral angiography. AJR Am J Roentgenol 1984; 142:247-53.

Citation:

Are the results of this single preventive or therapeutic trial valid?

Was the assignment of patients to treatments randomised?
Was the randomisation list concealed?

Were all patients who entered the trial accounted for at its conclusion?
Were they analysed in the groups to which they were randomised?

Were patients and clinicians kept 'blind' to which treatment was being received?

Aside from the experimental treatment, were the groups treated equally?

Were the groups similar at the start of the trial?

Are the valid results of this randomised trial important?

SAMPLE CALCULATIONS (see pp134–40 of *Evidence-based Medicine*)

Occurrence of diabetic neuropathy		Relative risk reduction (RRR)	Absolute risk reduction (ARR)	Number needed to treat (NNT)
Usual insulin control event rate (CER)	Intensive insulin experimental event rate (EER)	$\dfrac{CER - EER}{CER}$	CER – EER	1/ARR
9.6%	2.8%	$\dfrac{9.6\% - 2.8\%}{9.6\%}$ $= 71\%$	9.6% – 2.8% $= 6.8\%$	1/6.8% $= 15\text{pts}$

95% confidence interval (CI) on an NNT = 1 / (limits on the CI of its ARR) =

$$+/-1.96 \sqrt{\frac{CER \times (1\text{-}CER)}{\#\text{ of control pts.}} + \frac{EER \times (1\text{-}EER)}{\#\text{ of exper. pts.}}} = +/-1.96 \sqrt{\frac{0.96 \times 0.904}{730} + \frac{0.028 \times 0.972}{711}} = +/-2.4\%$$

Are the valid results of this randomised trial important?

YOUR CALCULATIONS

		Relative risk reduction (RRR)	Absolute risk reduction (ARR)	Number needed to treat (NNT)
CER	EER	$\dfrac{\text{CER} - \text{EER}}{\text{CER}}$	CER − EER	1/ARR

Can you apply this valid, important evidence about therapy in caring for your patient?

Do these results apply to your patient?

Is your patient so different from those in the trial
that its results can't help you?

*How great would the potential benefit of therapy
actually be for your individual patient?*

Method I: **f**	Risk of the outcome in your patient, relative to patients in the trial. Expressed as a decimal: _____ NNT/F = _____/_____ = _____ (NNT for patients like yours)
Method II: **1 / (PEER x RRR)**	Your patient's expected event rate if they received the control treatment: PEER: 1 / (PEER x RRR) = 1/_____ = _____ (NNT for patients like yours)

*Are your patient's values and preferences satisfied by
the regimen and its consequences?*

Do your patient and you have a clear assessment
of their values and preferences?

Are they met by this regimen and its consequences?

Additional notes

Citation: North American Symptomatic Carotid Endarterectomy Trial Collaborators: Beneficial effect of carotid endarterectomy in symptomatic patients with high-grade carotid stenosis. *New England Journal of Medicine* 1991; **325**: 445-53

Are the results of this single preventive or therapeutic trial valid?

Was the assignment of patients to treatments randomised?	**Yes.**
Was the randomisation list concealed?	**Yes.**
Were all patients who entered the trial accounted for at its conclusion?	**Yes.**
Were they analysed in the groups to which they were randomised?	**Yes.**
Were patients and clinicians kept 'blind' to which treatment was being received?	**No, but events went to 'blinded' adjudicators who decided whether and how severe a stroke had occurred.**
Aside from the experimental treatment, were the groups treated equally?	**Yes, with 'best medical Rx' including aspirin and vigorous antihypertensive therapy.**
Were the groups similar at the start of the trial?	**Yes.**

Are the valid results of this randomised trial important?

YOUR CALCULATIONS

Major stroke or death		Relative risk reduction (RRR)	Absolute risk reduction (ARR)	Number needed to treat (NNT)
CER	EER	$\dfrac{\text{CER} - \text{EER}}{\text{CER}}$	CER – EER	1/ARR
.181	**.080**	**56%** (28% to 84%)	**.101** (.050 to .152)	**10** (7 to 20)

95% confidence interval (CI) on an NNT = 1 / (limits on the CI of its ARR) =

$$+/\!-1.96 \sqrt{\frac{\text{CER} \times (1\text{-CER})}{\text{\# of control pts.}} + \frac{\text{EER} \times (1\text{-EER})}{\text{\# of exper. pts.}}} = +/\!-1.96 \sqrt{\frac{0.181 \times (1-0.181)}{331} + \frac{0.080 \times (1-0.080)}{328}}$$

Can you apply this valid, important evidence about therapy in caring for your patient?

Do these results apply to your patient?

Is your patient so different from those in the trial that its results can't help you?	**Similar.**

How great would the potential benefit of therapy actually be for your individual patient?

Method I: **f**	Risk of the outcome in your patient, relative to patients in the trial. Expressed as a decimal: **1** NNT/F = **10 / 1** = **10** (NNT for patients like yours)
Method II: **1 / (PEER x RRR)**	Your patient's expected event rate if they received the control treatment: PEER: 1 / (PEER x RRR) = 1/_____ = _____ (NNT for patients like yours)

Are your patient's values and preferences satisfied by the regimen and its consequences?

Do your patient and you have a clear assessment of their values and preferences?	**Needs to be addressed in each patient.**
Are they met by this regimen and its consequences?	**Needs to be addressed in each patient.**

Additional notes

1   Need to know the perioperative stroke rate for my surgeon.

2   Need to know the accuracy of carotid ultrasound at my hospital.

3   See also the European Carotid Surgery Trial (*Lancet* 1991;337:1235-43)

STROKE – CAROTID ENDARTERECTOMY REDUCES STROKE AND DEATH IN SYMPTOMATIC PTS WITH HIGH GRADE STENOSIS (NASCET).

Appraised by Sharon Straus and Dave Sackett; 26 Sept, 1996. Expiry date: 1999.

Clinical Bottom Line

In pts with recent hemispheric or retinal TIAs or nondisabling strokes, who have 70–99% stenosis of ipsilateral ICA, carotid endarterectomy decreases the risk of all stroke (NNT=7), major or fatal stroke (NNT=11), and major stroke or death (NNT=10) at 2 yrs.

Citation

NASCET Collaborators: Beneficial effect of carotid endarterectomy in symptomatic patients with high-grade carotid stenosis. *N Engl J Med* 1991; 325: 445–53.

Clinical Question

In patients with a recent cerebrovascular event, does carotid endarterectomy reduce the risk of subsequent major stroke and death?

Search Terms

'carotid endarterectomy' in *Best Evidence*.

The Study

1   Pts <80 yrs old, hemispheric TIA or monocular blindness <24 hrs or nondisabling stroke within previous 120 days in association with stenosis of 30–99% in ipsilateral ICA who were stratified into 2 strata – 30–69% and 70–99% stenosis.

2   Control group: (N=331) Medical care consisted of ASA (1300 mgs unless side effects), treatment of hypertension, hyperlipidemia or diabetes if appropriate. Follow up at 1,3,6,9,12 months and then q 4 months thereafter.

3   Experimental group: (N=328) Medical care and carotid endarterectomy. Follow up as with control group.

The Evidence

Outcome	Time to outcome	RRR	95% CI	ARR	95% CI	NNT	95% CI
Any stroke	2 yrs	54%	33% to 76%	0.150	0.090 to 0.210	7	5 to 11
Major or fatal stroke	2 yrs	72%	40% to 100%	0.094	0.052 to 0.136	11	7 to 19
Any major stroke or death	2 yrs	56%	28% to 84%	0.101	0.050 to 0.152	10	7 to 20

Comments

1   Trial stopped early in pts with high grade stenosis because of evidence of efficacy of surgery.

2   No patient lost to follow up and no pt withdrawn.

3   Extrapolation to your hospital – if your hospital's perioperative risk of major stroke and death exceeds 2.1%, benefit of surgery starts to fall and if the rate of major complications approaches 10% the benefit vanishes entirely.

PART A Critical appraisal of a clinical article about the diagnosis of anaemia

You admit a 75-year old woman with community-acquired pneumonia. She responds nicely to appropriate antibiotics but her haemoglobin remains at 100 g/l with a mean cell volume of 80. Her peripheral blood smear shows hypochromia, but she is otherwise well and is on no incriminating medications. You contact her GP and find out that her haemoglobin was 105 g/l six months ago. She has never been investigated for anaemia. You discuss this patient with your registrar and debate the use of ferritin in the diagnosis of iron deficiency anaemia. You admit to yourself that you are unsure how to interpret a ferritin result and about how precise and accurate ferritin is for diagnosing iron deficiency anaemia.

You therefore form the question: 'In an elderly woman with hypochromic, microcytic anaemia, can a low ferritin diagnose iron deficiency anaemia?' You order a ferritin and head for the library (10 days later it comes back at 40 µg/l).

Searching *Best Evidence* on Disk with the single word 'ferritin' yielded a very encouraging meta-analysis of 55 studies and a nice individual study, but your library didn't carry either journal. You perform a MEDLINE search using the MeSH terms 'ferritin' and ('sensitivity and specificity') and find an article on diagnosing iron deficiency anaemia in the elderly published in a journal that your library does receive (*Am J Med* (1990) **88:** 205-9).

Read this article and decide:
1 Are the results of this diagnostic article valid?
2 Are the valid results of this diagnostic study important?
3 Can you apply this valid, important evidence about a diagnostic test in caring for your patient?

If you want to read some strategies for answering these sorts of questions, look at pp 81–84; 118–128; and 159–163 in *Evidence-based Medicine*.

PART B Asking answerable clinical questions

1 We will illustrate the importance, strategies and tactics of formulating clinical questions and work with you on Parts 3–4 of the question.

2 Participants will break up into groups of two, discuss patients they cared for in the previous week, and generate questions they think are important concerning their patients' therapy, diagnosis and prognosis.

3 In larger groups, we will review and refine the questions and then keep track of them as possible questions to use in later sessions devoted to searching for the best evidence.

Diagnosis of Iron-Deficiency Anemia in the Elderly

Gordon H. Guyatt, M.D., Christopher Patterson, M.D., Mahmoud Ali, M.D., Joel Singer, Ph.D., Mark Levine, M.D., Irene Turpie, M.D., Ralph Meyer, M.D., Hamilton, Ontario, Canada

PURPOSE: To determine the value of serum ferritin, mean cell volume, transferrin saturation, and free erythrocyte protoporphyrin in the diagnosis of iron-deficiency anemia in the elderly.

PATIENTS AND METHODS: We prospectively studied consecutive eligible and consenting anemic patients over the age of 65 years, who underwent blood tests and bone marrow aspiration. The study consisted of 259 inpatients and outpatients at two community hospitals in whom a complete blood count processed by the hospital laboratory demonstrated previously undiagnosed anemia (men: hemoglobin level less than 12 g/dL; women: hemoglobin level less than 11.0 g/dL).

RESULTS: Thirty-six percent of our patients had no demonstrable marrow iron and were classified as being iron-deficient. The serum ferritin was the best test for distinguishing those with iron deficiency from those who were not iron-deficient. No other test added clinically important information. The likelihood ratios associated with the serum ferritin level were as follows: greater than 100 μg/L, 0.13; greater than 45 μg/L but less than or equal to 100 μg/L, 0.46; greater than 18 μg/L but less than or equal to 45 μg/L, 3.12; and less than or equal to 18 μg/L, 41.47. These results indicate that values up to 45 μg/L increase the likelihood of iron deficiency, whereas values over 45 μg/L decrease the likelihood of iron deficiency. Seventy-two percent of those who were not iron-deficient had serum ferritin values greater than 100 μg/L, and in populations with a prevalence of iron deficiency of less than 40%, values of greater than 100 μg/L reduce the probability of iron deficiency to under 10%. Fifty-five percent of the iron-deficient patients had serum ferritin values of less than 18 μg/L, and in populations with a prevalence of iron deficiency of greater than 20%, values of less than 18 μg/L increase the probability of iron deficiency to over 95%.

CONCLUSION: In a general geriatric medical population such as ours, with a prevalence of iron deficiency of 36%, appropriate use of serum ferritin determination would establish or refute a diagnosis of iron deficiency without a bone marrow aspiration in 70% of the patients.

Anemia is an extremely common problem in the elderly, and next to anemia of chronic disease, iron deficiency is the most common cause. Iron-deficiency anemia is important to diagnose because appropriate iron therapy may improve symptoms, inappropriate iron therapy may cause clinically important side effects, and iron deficiency may be a marker for occult gastrointestinal pathology.

Although bone marrow aspiration provides a definitive diagnosis of iron-deficiency anemia, the value of less invasive tests of iron stores in general populations has been well established [1–9]. Serum ferritin and transferrin saturation are the tests most commonly used. Because bone marrow aspiration can be painful and is more expensive than laboratory tests, the procedure is often reserved for patients in whom the diagnosis remains in doubt after noninvasive test results are available.

Our interest in the investigation of iron deficiency in the elderly was stimulated by a clinical impression that application of cutoff points for laboratory tests for the diagnosis of iron deficiency derived from younger populations was misleading in a geriatric population. There are a number of reasons why results found in younger populations may not apply to the elderly. The iron-binding capacity decreases with aging [10,11], and is affected by factors such as malnutrition and chronic disease, which have a higher prevalence in the elderly [12]. Serum ferritin levels increase with aging [13], and may be elevated by acute and chronic inflammatory conditions [14,15]. One small study has suggested that measurements of transferrin saturation and serum ferritin in elderly anemic patients with and without iron deficiency differ significantly from those found in younger patients [16]. These problems have led to varying recommendations regarding the interpretation of results of noninvasive tests of iron stores in the elderly [16–18].

There are other reasons why further study of the diagnosis of anemia is warranted. First, investigations to date have generally used a single cut-point, and reported on the sensitivity and specificity of the tests. This approach discards valuable information. Use of multiple cut-points, with determination of likelihood ratios associated with each range of results, provides additional information for the clinician [19]. Second, statistically reliable determination of the best single test, and whether additional useful information could

From the Department of Medicine (GHG, CP, MA, ML, IT, RM), the Department of Clinical Epidemiology and Biostatistics (GHG, ML), and the Department of Family Practice (JS), McMaster University, Hamilton, Ontario, Canada. This work was supported in part by the Ontario Ministry of Health. Dr. Guyatt is a Career Scientist of the Ontario Ministry of Health. Requests for reprints should be addressed to Gordon H. Guyatt, M.D., Department of Clinical Epidemiology and Biostatistics, McMaster University Health Sciences Centre, Room 2C12; 1200 Main Street West, Hamilton, Ontario, Canada, L8N 3Z5. Manuscript submitted July 13, 1989, and accepted in revised form November 14, 1989.

Current addresses: Department of Medicine, Chedoke Hospital, Hamilton, Ontario, Canada (CP); Department of Pathology, St. Joseph's Hospital, Hamilton, Ontario, Canada (MA); Department of Medicine, St. Joseph's Hospital, Hamilton, Ontario, Canada (IT); Department of Family Medicine, McMaster University Health Sciences Centre, Hamilton, Ontario, Canada (JS); and Department of Medicine, Henderson General Hospital, Hamilton, Ontario, Canada (ML, RM).

TABLE I

Reasons For Exclusion of Patients Found To Be Anemic on at Least One Hemoglobin Determination

Reason for Exclusion	Number of Patients Excluded
Patient judged too ill, demented, or terminal	212
Patient or family refused consent for bone marrow aspiration	200
Not anemic on second hemoglobin determination	200
Recent transfusion	152
Previous bone marrow aspiration had revealed diagnosis	108
Institutionalized	95
Miscellaneous	108
Total	**1,075**

TABLE II

Final Primary Diagnosis of Anemia

Diagnosis	Number of Patients
Iron-deficiency anemia	94
Anemia of chronic disease	113
Megaloblastic anemia	21
Multiple myeloma	4
Sideroblastic anemia	3
Dysmyeloplastic	3
Other*	21
Total	**259**

* Includes patients with leukemia, hemolytic anemia, hypoplastic and aplastic marrow, renal failure, and hypothyroidism, and those with inadequate information for definitive diagnosis.

be gained from performing a second or third test, has seldom been investigated. Third, other tests (including the free erythrocyte protoporphyrin) have been suggested as being potentially useful in confirming the diagnosis of iron-deficiency anemia, but have not been adequately studied.

Because of the frequency of anemia in the elderly, and because of the difficulties in performing bone marrow aspirations in all anemic patients, we believed it important to determine the accuracy of less invasive laboratory tests commonly used to assess iron stores. Our criterion or gold standard for the diagnosis of iron deficiency was the results of the bone marrow aspiration.

PATIENTS AND METHODS

Consecutive patients over the age of 65 years presenting to Chedoke Hospital in Hamilton, Ontario, between January 1984 and March 1988 with anemia (in men, hemoglobin 12.0 g/dL or less on two consecutive occasions; in women, 11.0 g/dL or less) were identified through the hospital laboratory. An additional much smaller group of patients admitted to St. Joseph's Hospital in Hamilton under one of the co-investigators and meeting study criteria were also included. We excluded institutionalized patients, those with recent blood transfusions or documented acute blood loss, or those whose participation in the study was judged unethical by their attending physician (for reasons such as impending death or severe dementia). Detailed criteria for definition of "too ill," "impending

death," or "severe dementia" were not established. Rather, we relied on physician judgment in these areas. Similarly, we relied on physicians for the appropriate level of encouragement to patient participation when obtaining informed consent.

All patients had the following laboratory tests: hemoglobin, mean red cell volume (MCV), red cell distribution width (RDW), serum iron, iron-binding capacity, serum ferritin, and red cell protoporphyrin. The complete blood count was carried out using a Coulter S +IV™ (Coulter Electronics, Miami, Florida). Serum iron and iron-binding capacity were measured according to the methods of the International Committee for Standardization in Haematology [20]. Serum ferritin was determined using a radioimmunoassay described in detail previously [21]. Red cell protoporphyrin was measured using a previously described micromethod [22]. A bone marrow aspiration was undertaken and the findings were interpreted by a hematologist (M.A.) who was unaware of the results of the laboratory tests. The bone marrow slides were air-dried, fixed with methanol, and stained with Prussian blue [23]. Results of the first 65 marrow aspirations were also interpreted by a second hematologist (also unaware of the laboratory test findings), and discrepancies resolved by consensus. The results of the aspiration were classified as iron absent, reduced, present, or increased. After interpreting the marrow aspiration results, the hematologist reviewed all relevant clinical information and made a final decision regarding the cause(s) of the anemia. Anemia of chronic disease was diagnosed when the iron present in the reticuloendothelial cells (fragments) was increased and the number of sideroblasts (red cells containing iron granules) was decreased. The increase in reticuloendothelial iron was defined as iron granules covering 50% of all the fragments observed, and a decrease in sideroblasts was confirmed when iron granules were present in less than 20% of the red cells.

Statistical Methods

Receiver operating characteristic (ROC) curves for each test were generated. The area under the curves was compared using the method of Hanley and McNeil [24]. Since the ROC curves in this study were all generated from the same cohort of patients, we used the correction factor, which reflects the correlation between the tests [25]. Using the same cut-points, likelihood ratios for each category were calculated.

To determine the independent contribution of each test to the diagnosis, and whether a combination of tests could improve diagnostic accuracy, stepwise logistic regression procedures were used. The status of iron stores (present or absent) was used as the dependent variable, and the values of the diagnostic tests (dichotomized using the cut-point that maximized accuracy) as the independent variables.

Chance-corrected agreement between the two hematologists who interpreted the marrow aspiration results was calculated using a weighted kappa, with quadratic weights.

RESULTS

Aside from providing more precise estimates of the likelihood ratios, inclusion of 25 patients from St. Joseph's Hospital had no systematic effect on the results of any analysis. Thus, these patients will not be identi-

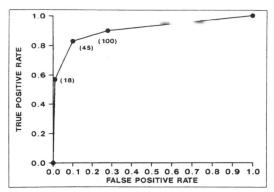

Figure 1. ROC curve for serum ferritin.

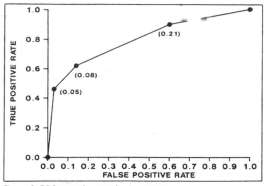

Figure 2. ROC curve for transferrin saturation.

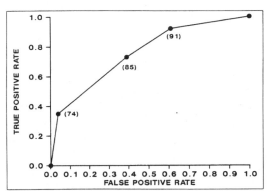

Figure 3. ROC curve for mean cell volume.

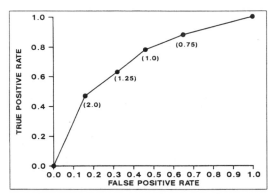

Figure 4. ROC curve for free erythrocyte protoporphyrin.

fied separately in the presentation of the results that follows.

A total of 1,334 patients over 65 years with anemia was identified. Of these, 259 proved eligible, participated in the study, and underwent bone marrow aspiration. Seventy-six participants were outpatients, and 183 were inpatients. Of the 259 bone marrow aspirates from the patients, 235 were interpretable (the quality being too poor in the others). The reasons for exclusion of anemic patients are presented in **Table I**. Most of the patients who recently received transfusions were postoperative patients, a large proportion of whom (at a hospital with a very busy orthopedic service) had undergone total hip replacement or had a recent hip fracture.

The mean age (± SD) of the participating patients was 79.7 ± 7.62 years; 119 (46%) were men. The mean hemoglobin level was 9.81 g/dL (± 1.39); 52.1% of the patients had a hemoglobin level less than 10.0 g/dL. A very wide variety of illnesses were not directly related to the anemia. Seventy-two patients had no medical diagnosis other than anemia (and its cause); 72 had one other diagnosis; 67 had two other diagnoses; 34 had three other diagnoses; and 14 had more than three other diagnoses. The most common medical diagnoses (aside from anemia), and the number of patients affected, were as follows: early dementia, 25; congestive heart failure, 25; chronic airflow limitation, 17; rheumatoid arthritis, 17; osteoarthritis, 14; pneumonia, 13.

The final diagnoses of anemia are presented in **Table II**. The weighted kappa-quantifying chance-corrected agreement for the 65 marrow aspirates that were interpreted by two hematologists was 0.84.

Figures 1 to **4** present the ROC curves for serum ferritin, transferrin saturation, MCV, and red cell protoporphyrin. Because, through administrative error and lost samples, all tests were not conducted in all subjects, the number of patients available for each analysis varied, and was sometimes less than 235. Examination of the ROC curves revealed that serum ferritin performed far better than any of the other tests. This was confirmed by the statistical analysis, which showed that the area under the ROC curves was 0.91, 0.79, 0.78, and 0.72 (respectively), for the four tests. Although the difference between the serum ferritin and the other three tests was statistically significant (p ≤0.001 in each case), any differences seen in the other four curves can easily be explained by chance (p ≥0.1).

Likelihood ratios for the four tests are presented in **Table III**. Consistent with the ROC curves, serum ferritin showed a far greater discriminative power than the other tests.

Likelihood ratios for RDW for distinguishing those with iron deficiency from those with anemia of chronic disease were examined. The likelihood ratios for RDW 0 to 15, 15 to 19, and greater than 19 were 0.39, 1.31, and 1.90, respectively. Ferritin proved a far more powerful predictor for differentiating iron deficiency from

March 1990   The American Journal of Medicine   Volume 88   207

Session 2 – Diagnosis & asking answerable clinical questions

TABLE III

Likelihood Ratios

Interval	Number Iron-Deficient	Number Not Iron-Deficient	Likelihood Ratio
Ferritin			
>100	8	108	0.13
>45 ≤ 100	7	27	0.46
>18 ≤ 45	23	13	3.12
≤18	47	2	41.47
Total	85	150	
Transferrin saturation			
>0.21	9	55	0.28
>0.8 ≤ 0.21	23	70	0.57
>0.05 ≤ 0.08	14	17	1.43
≤0.05	38	4	16.51
Total	84	146	
Mean cell volume			
>95	2	32	0.11
>91 − ≤ 95	5	26	0.34
>85 − ≤ 91	16	44	0.64
>74 − ≤ 85	32	42	1.35
≤74	30	6	8.82
Total	85	150	
Red cell protoporphyrin			
≥ 0 ≤ 0.75	10	53	0.34
>0.75 ≤ 0.1	8	28	0.51
>1 − ≤ 1.25	9	21	0.77
>1.25 ≤ 2	17	24	1.26
>2	40	24	2.98
Total	84	150	

TABLE IV

Likelihood Ratios from Logistic Regression Analysis

Interval	Number Iron-Deficient	Number Not Iron-Deficient	Likelihood Ratio
Ferritin			
Ferritin negative*†, transferrin saturation negative‡	13	126	0.18
Only ferritin positive	33	10	5.72
Ferritin positive, transferrin saturation positive	33	1	57.23
Total	79	137	

* Only four cases were serum ferritin-negative and transferrin saturation-positive.
† Cut-point for serum ferritin was 45 μg/L.
‡ Cut-point for transferrin saturation was 0.08.

TABLE V

Post-Test Probability of Iron Deficiency Given Varying Pre-Test Probabilities and Results of Serum Ferritin Determinations

Serum ferritin result (μg/L)	Pre-Test Probability Low (5%–20%)	Intermediate (40%–60%)	High (80%–95%)	Study Population (36%)
>100	0.6–3	8–16	34–71	7
45–100	2–10	24–41	39–90	21
18–45	14–44	68–82	93–98	64
<18	69–91	97–98	99–99.9	96

anemia of chronic disease, with likelihood ratios ranging from 0.05 to infinity. Finally, RDW added little to the predictive power of serum ferritin.

In the logistic regression model, ferritin was the best predictor of bone marrow iron stores. The only test that explained a statistically significant additional portion of the variance was the transferrin saturation. Using a cutoff of 45 μg/L for ferritin and 0.08 for transferrin saturation, likelihood ratios generated by using a combination of the tests are presented in **Table IV**. Little is gained by this model in comparison to serum ferritin: likelihood ratios greater than 1 are slightly higher, but the likelihood ratio less than 1 is not as low as the value obtained with a serum ferritin level of greater than 100 μg/L. Of patients with serum ferritin values of 18 to 100 μg/L, seven had transferrin saturation values of less than 0.05. All seven of these patients proved to be iron-deficient.

Other studies have reported elevated serum ferritin levels in patients with liver disease and inflammatory diseases, particularly rheumatoid arthritis [2,3,5,6,8,14,15]. Of the five patients with liver disease who were iron-deficient, three had serum ferritin values less than 18 μg/L. Of the six iron-deficient subjects with rheumatoid arthritis, five had a serum ferritin level less than 18 μg/L. Therefore, in our study, patients with liver disease or rheumatoid arthritis appeared to behave in a manner similar to that in the rest of the population. However, the numbers of patients with these conditions were insufficient to permit strong inference regarding the issue of differences among subgroups.

COMMENTS

Previous studies in younger subjects have consistently shown the usefulness of serum ferritin in the diagnosis of iron-deficiency anemia, and suggested that serum ferritin is more powerful than other blood tests [1–9]. Our results are consistent with these findings: in elderly patients with anemia, serum ferritin determination is by far the best test for diagnosis of iron deficiency. Other tests add only limited information in the diagnosis.

The MCV is ordinarily available with the complete blood count, and could thus influence the estimate of the probability of iron deficiency prior to ordering of other tests. However, in our population, even MCV values of less than 74 were not invariably associated with iron deficiency, and in many of the patients with iron deficiency the anemia was not microcytic. Only 6% of those with an MCV greater than 95 had iron deficiency; therefore, a very large MCV can be interpreted as virtually excluding iron deficiency.

The likelihood ratios for the possible ranges of results of serum ferritin determinations are presented in Table III. Previous studies in uncomplicated anemia have led to recommended cutoff points between normal and abnormal of 12 to 20 μg/L [1–9]. Using this approach, any value above 20 μg/L would be treated as a negative test result and as decreasing the likelihood of the patient having iron deficiency. In fact, in our population, ferritin values between 18 and 45 μg/L reflected an increase in the likelihood of iron deficiency (Table III), and the optimal cutoff in terms of maximizing accuracy was 45 μg/L (Figure 1). This result likely reflects the fact that serum ferritin levels increase with age [13]. It may also reflect the high preva-lence of chronic disease in the elderly, although only a small proportion of our population had inflammatory conditions thought to be associated with increased lev-els of serum ferritin.

Although these results might lead to the conclusion that a higher cutoff for serum ferritin should be used in the elderly, more information is to be gained by using multiple cut-points. The clinical usefulness of the likelihood ratios associated within different re-sults of serum ferritin is illustrated in **Table V**. Table V examines four different scenarios: patients with low (5% to 20%), intermediate (40% to 60%), and high (80% to 95%) pre-test probability or prevalence of iron defi-ciency as an explanation for their anemia, as well as the population of the current study (in whom the prev-alence of iron deficiency was 36%). The power of the serum ferritin level is made evident by examining the patients with intermediate probability, in whom the post-test probability of iron deficiency decreases to 8% to 16% if the serum ferritin level is greater than 100 μg/L, while a result of less than 18 μg/L increases the likelihood of iron deficiency to greater than 97%. Let us assume a physician is willing to diagnose a patient with a probability of 10% or less as not having iron-deficiency anemia, and a patient with a probability of 90% or more as having iron deficiency, without per-forming a bone marrow examination. Under these cir-cumstances, a serum ferritin value of greater than 45 μg/L will obviate the necessity of a bone marrow aspi-ration in all patients with low prior probability; and a result of less than 18 μg/L in those with an intermedi-ate prior probability, or less than 45 μg/L in those with a high prior probability, secures the diagnosis of iron deficiency.

The results depicted in the last column of Table IV suggest that, for clinicians dealing with populations similar to the one included in the present study, pa-tients with values greater than 100 μg/L can be treated as not having iron deficiency, patients with values of less than 18 μg/L can be treated as having iron defi-ciency, and a bone marrow aspiration is necessary for diagnosis in those with intermediate values. Using this approach would lead to a diagnosis of iron deficiency in 21% of the patients, and exclusion of iron deficiency in 49%. Thus, bone marrow aspiration would be re-quired in only 30%.

The present study has a number of strengths in comparison to previous investigations of the useful-ness of laboratory tests in the diagnosis of iron defi-ciency. The sample represents a group of consecutive elderly patients presenting with anemia. We demon-strated the reproducibility of the interpretation of re-sults of bone marrow aspiration, the procedure was undertaken in all patients, and the findings were inter-preted by a hematologist unaware of the results of the laboratory investigations. We can therefore be confi-dent of our conclusion that serum ferritin is the one peripheral blood test useful in the diagnosis of iron-deficiency anemia in the elderly; that the results

should be interpreted differently from serum ferritin results in younger patients; and that when the infor-mation from the test is optimally utilized (by means of multi-level likelihood ratios), the test is extremely powerful in the diagnosis of iron-deficiency anemia.

ACKNOWLEDGMENT

We thank the following individuals for their help in data collection and preparation of this manuscript: Dr. Anne Benger for help with interpretation of bone marrow aspirates; and Sue Halcrow, Sandi Harper, Jenny Whyte, and Debbie Maddock for help with data collection, data processing, and manuscript preparation.

REFERENCES

1. Beck JR, Gibbons AB, Cornwell G, et al: Multivariate approach to predictive diagnosis of bone-marrow iron stores. Am J Clin Pathol 1979; 70: S665–S670.
2. Sheehan RG, Newton MJ, Frenkel EP: Evaluation of a packaged kit assay of serum ferritin and application to clinical diagnosis of selected anemias. Am J Clin Pathol 1978; 70: 79–84.
3. Krause JR, Stolc V: Serum ferritin and bone marrow biopsy iron stores. Am J Clin Pathol 1980; 74: S461–S464.
4. Ali MAM, Luxton AW, Walker WHC: Serum ferritin concentration and bone mar-row iron stores: a prospective study. Can Med Assoc J 1978; 118: 945–946.
5. Mazza J, Barr RM, McDonald JWD, Valberg LS: Usefulness of the serum ferritin concentration in the detection of iron deficiency in a general hospital. Can Med Assoc J 1978; 119: 884–886.
6. Sorbie J, Valberg LS, Corbett WEN, Ludwig J: Serum ferritin, cobalt excretion and body iron status. Can Med Assoc J 1975; 112: 1173–1178.
7. Addison GM, Beamish MR, Hales CN, et al: An immunoradiometric assay for ferritin in the serum of normal subjects and patients with iron deficiency and iron overload. J Clin Pathol 1972; 25: 326–329.
8. Lipschitz DA, Cook JD, Finch CA: A clinical evaluation of serum ferritin as an index of iron stores. N Engl J Med 1974; 290: 1213–1216.
9. Walsh JR, Fredrickson M: Serum ferritin, free erythrocyte protoporphyrin, and urinary iron excretion in patients with iron disorders. Am J Med Sci 1977; 273: 293–300.
10. Pirie R: The influence of age upon serum iron in normal subjects. J Clin Pathol 1952; 5: 10–15.
11. Yip R, Johnson C, Dallman PR: Age-related changes in laboratory values used in the diagnosis of anemia and iron deficiency. Am J Clin Nutr 1984; 39: 427–436.
12. Powell DEB, Thomas JH: The iron binding capacity of serum in elderly hospital patients. Gerontol Clin (Basel) 1969; 11: 36–47.
13. Loria A, Hershko C, Konij N: Serum ferritin in an elderly population. J Gerontol 1979; 34: 521–525.
14. Nelson R, Chawla M, Connolly P, Laporte J: Ferritin as an index of bone marrow iron stores. South Med J 1978; 71: 1482–1484.
15. Bentley DP, Williams P: Serum ferritin concentration as an index of storage iron in rheumatoid arthritis. J Clin Pathol 1974; 27: 786–788.
16. Patterson C, Turpie ID, Benger AM: Assessment of iron stores in anemic geriat-ric patients. J Am Geriatr Soc 1985; 33: 746–767.
17. Awad MO, Berford AV, Grindulis KA, et al: Factors affecting the serum iron-binding capacity in the elderly. Gerontology 1982; 28: 125–131.
18. Lynch SR, Finch CA, Monsen ER, et al: Iron status of elderly Americans. Am J Clin Nutr 1982; 36: 1032–1045.
19. Department of Clinical Epidemiology and Biostatistics, McMaster University: Interpretation of diagnostic data: how to do it with simple maths. Can Med Assoc J 1983; 129: 22–29.
20. International Committee for Standardization in Haematology: The measure-ment of total iron and unsaturated iron binding capacity in serum. Br J Haematol 1978; 38: 281–287.
21. Luxton AW, Walker WHC, Gauldie J, Ali MAM, Pelletier C: A radioimmunoassay for serum ferritin. Clin Chem 1977; 23: 683–689.
22. Piomelli S, Young P, Gay G: A micro method for free erythrocyte protoporphy-rin: the FEP test. J Lab Clin Med 1973; 81: 932–940.
23. Dacie SV, Lewis SM: Practical hematology, 6th ed. New York: Churchill Living-stone, 1984; 107–109.
24. Hanley JA, McNeil BJ: The meaning and use of the area under a receiver operating characteristic (ROC) curve. Radiology 1982; 143: 29–36.
25. Hanley JA, McNeil BJ: A method of comparing the areas under receiver operat-ing characteristic curves derived from the same cases. Radiology 1983; 148: 839–843.

Citation:

Are the results of this diagnostic study valid?

Was there an independent, blind comparison with a
reference ('gold') standard of diagnosis?

Was the diagnostic test evaluated in an appropriate
spectrum of patients (like those in whom it would
be used in practice)?

Was the reference standard applied regardless of
the diagnostic test result?

Are the valid results of this diagnostic study important?

SAMPLE CALCULATIONS (see p120 of *Evidence-based Medicine*)

		Target disorder (iron deficiency anaemia)		Totals
		Present	Absent	
Diagnostic test result	Positive (<65 mmol/L)	731 a	270 b	a+b 1001
(serum ferritin)	Negative (≥65 mmol/L)	78 c	1500 d	c+d 1578
	Totals	809 a+c	1770 b+d	a+b+c+d 2579

Sensitivity = a/(a+c) = 731/809 = 90%

Specificity = d/(b+d) = 1500/1770 = 85%

Likelihood Ratio for a positive test result = LR+=sens/(1-spec)=90%/15%=6

Likelihood Ratio for a negative test result=LR-=(1-sens)/spec=10%/85%=0.12

Positive Predictive Value = a/(a+b) = 731/1001 = 73%

Negative Predictive Value = d/(c+d) = 1500/1578 = 95%

Pre-test Probability (prevalence) = (a+c)/(a+b+c+d) = 809/2579 = 32%

Pre-test-odds = prevalence/(1-prevalence) = 31%/69% = 0.45

Post-test odds = Pre-test odds x Likelihood Ratio

Post-test Probability = Post-test odds/(Post-test odds + 1)

Are the valid results of this diagnostic study important?

YOUR CALCULATIONS

		Target disorder		Totals
		Present	**Absent**	
Diagnostic test result	Positive	a	b	a+b
	Negative	c	d	c+d
	Totals	a+c	b+d	a+b+c+d

Sensitivity = a/(a+c) =   Specificity = d/(b+d) =

Likelihood Ratio for a positive test result = LR+=sens/(1-spec)=

Likelihood Ratio for a negative test result=LR-=(1-sens)/spec=

Positive Predictive Value = a/(a+b) =   Negative Predictive Value = d/(c+d) =

Pre-test Probability (prevalence) = (a+c)/(a+b+c+d) =

Pre-test-odds = prevalence/(1-prevalence) =

Post-test odds = Pre-test odds x Likelihood Ratio =

Post-test Probability = Post-test odds/(Post-test odds + 1) =

Can you apply this valid, important evidence about a diagnostic test in caring for your patient?

Is the diagnostic test available, affordable, accurate, and precise in your setting?

Can you generate a clinically sensible estimate of your patient's pre-test probability (from practice data, personal experience, the report itself, or clinical speculation)?

Will the resulting post-test probabilities affect your management and help your patient? (Could it move you across a test-treatment threshold? Would your patient be a willing partner in carrying it out?)

Would the consequences of the test help your patient?

Additional notes

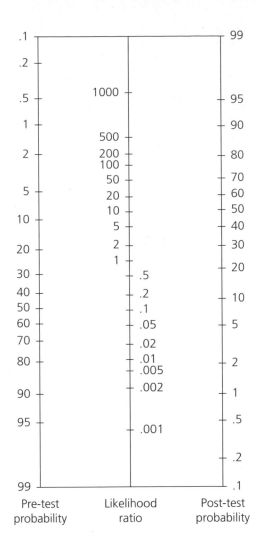

Anchor a straight-edge along the left edge of the nomogram at your patient's pre-test probability and pivot it until it intersects the likelihood ratio for your patient's diagnostic test result. It will intersect the right edge of the nomogram at your patient's post-test probability. Test 1: for a likelihood ratio of 1, pre-test and post-test probabilities should be identical. Test 2: for a pre-test probability of 30% and a likelihood ratio of 5, the post-test probability is just under 70%.

Adapted from Fagan TJ (1975) Nomogram for Bayes' theorem. *N Engl J Med.* **293**: 257.

Citation: Guyatt GH, Patterson C, Ali M, Singer J, *et al.* (1990) Diagnosis of iron-deficiency anemia in the elderly. *Am J Med* 1990; 88: 205-9

Are the results of this diagnostic study valid?

Was there an independent, blind comparison with a reference ('gold') standard of diagnosis?	**Yes, they underwent bone-marrow aspirations.**
Was the diagnostic test evaluated in an appropriate spectrum of patients (like those in whom it would be used in practice)?	**Yes.**
Was the reference standard applied regardless of the diagnostic test result?	**Yes.**

Are the valid results of this diagnostic study important?

Ferritin	Iron deficiency	No iron deficiency	Likelihood ratio
≤45	70/85	15/150	8.2
>45≤100	7/85	27/150	0.44
>100	8/85	108/150	0.13
Totals	85	150	

● **For pre-test probabilities in the 30–70% range, a ferritin ≤45 would be very helpful, yielding post-test probabilities of 78–95% (in the latter case, a SpPin[1]).**

● **In that same pre-test probability range, a ferritin >100 would yield post-test probabilities of 5–23% (in the former case, a SnNout[2]).**

● **So it can give quite important results.**

[1]When a diagnostic test has a very high **Sp**ecificity, a **P**ositive result Rules-**In** the diagnosis.

[2]When a diagnostic test has a very high **Se**nsitivity, a **N**egative result Rules-**Out** the diagnosis.

Can you apply this valid, important evidence about a diagnostic test in caring for your patient?

Is the diagnostic test available, affordable, accurate, and precise in your setting?	**Needs to be assessed in each setting.**
Can you generate a clinically sensible estimate of your patient's pre-test probability (from practice data, personal experience, the report itself, or clinical speculation)?	**Approximately 30%.**
Will the resulting post-test probabilities affect your management and help your patient? (Could it move you across a test-treatment threshold? Would your patient be a willing partner in carrying it out?)	**Her result of 40 brings her post-test probability to 78%, certainly high enough for you to want to investigate her for causes of anaemia (GI loss, etc.).**
Would the consequences of the test help your patient?	**Yes, if it led to a reversible cause. But this would have to be weighed against early detection of an untreatable cause, e.g. cancer, that would simply take away 'healthy' time. The options would need to be discussed with your patient.**

Additional notes

1 An excellent overview of 55 studies of lab tests for Fe-deficient anaemia: Guyatt *et al*. (1992) *J Gen Intern Med.* **7**: 145–53 (with a correction on page 423).

A LIKELIHOOD RATIO NOMOGRAM

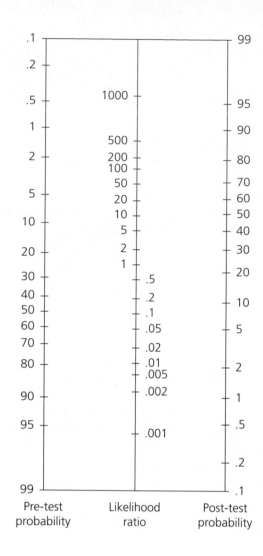

Pre-test probability   Likelihood ratio   Post-test probability

Anchor a straight-edge along the left edge of the nomogram at your patient's pre-test probability and pivot it until it intersects the likelihood ratio for your patient's diagnostic test result. It will intersect the right edge of the nomogram at your patient's post-test probability. Test 1: for a likelihood ratio of 1, pre-test and post-test probabilities should be identical. Test 2: for a pre-test probability of 30% and a likelihood ratio of 5, the post-test probability is just under 70%.

Adapted from Fagan TJ (1975) Nomogram for Bayes' theorem. *N Engl J Med.* **293**: 257.

Clinical Bottom Line
In community-dwelling elderly medical patients in whom iron deficiency anaemia is suspected, serum ferritin is a valid, precise diagnostic test.

Citation
Guyatt GH, Patterson C, Ali M *et al*. (1990) Diagnosis of iron-deficiency anemia in the elderly. *Am J Med* **88:**205-9.

Clinical Question
In a patient with anaemia, can a low serum ferritin be used to diagnose iron deficiency anaemia in the elderly?

Search Terms
'ferritin' and ('sensitivity and specificity')

The Study
1   Gold Standard – bone marrow aspiration.

2   Study setting – consecutive pts over the age of 65 who were admitted with anaemia to a university-affiliated hospital in Canada.

The Evidence

Ferritin	Iron deficiency	No iron deficiency	Likelihood ratio
≤45	70/85	15/150	8.2
>45≤100	7/85	27/150	0.44
>100	8/85	108/150	0.13
Totals	85	150	

Comments
1   Excluded pts from institutions and pts who were 'too ill' or had 'severe dementia' although these were not defined.

2   Weighted kappa for bone marrow interpretation by 2 haematologists was 0.84.

3   Low values can SpPin, and high values can SnNout.

4   Also see the meta-analysis in *J Gen Intern Med* 1992;**7:**145-53. (with a correction on page 423).

Appraised by Sharon Straus, Nov 1996.
Expiry date: 1998.

Diagnosis & asking answerable clinical questions

PART A Critical appraisal of a clinical article about the diagnosis of pulmonary embolism

A 55-year old woman with shortness of breath and pleuritic chest pain is readmitted one week after discharge following a cholecystectomy. She is on no medications and her past medical history is unremarkable. Physical exam is also unremarkable except for her nicely healing cholecystectomy scar. Lab results reveal a decreased pO_2 of 6 kPa (60 mm Hg) on room air and an elevated A-a gradient.

You suspect a PE and your Registrar/Senior Resident tells you to anticoagulate the patient and to order a ventilation/perfusion (V/Q) lung scan, which is reported as 'high probability'. You admit to yourself that you don't quite understand the usefulness of lung scans in diagnosing pulmonary embolism and decide to brush up on the literature.

You form the clinical question: 'In patients with clinically suspected pulmonary embolism, how sensitive and specific is a "high-probability" V/Q scan?' You perform a MEDLINE literature search using the text words: 'pulmonary embolism', 'high-probability' and 'lung scans' and find the PIOPED article which looks relevant. (*JAMA* (1990); **263:** 2753-9).

Read the article and decide:
1 Are the results of this diagnosis study valid?
2 Are the results of this diagnosis study important?
3 Can you apply this valid, important evidence about a diagnostic test in caring for your patient?

If you want to read some strategies for answering these sorts of questions, look at pp 81–84; 118–128; and 159–163 in *Evidence-based Medicine*.

PART B — Asking answerable clinical questions

1 We illustrate the importance, strategies and tactics of formulating clinical questions and work with you on Parts 3–4 of the question.

2 Participants will break up into groups of two, discuss patients they cared for in the previous week, and generate questions they think are important concerning their patients' therapy, diagnosis and prognosis.

3 In larger groups, we will review and refine the questions and then keep track of them as possible questions to use in later sessions devoted to searching for the best evidence.

Original Contributions

Value of the Ventilation/Perfusion Scan in Acute Pulmonary Embolism

Results of the Prospective Investigation of Pulmonary Embolism Diagnosis (PIOPED)

The PIOPED Investigators

To determine the sensitivities and specificities of ventilation/perfusion lung scans for acute pulmonary embolism, a random sample of 933 of 1493 patients was studied prospectively. Nine hundred thirty-one underwent scintigraphy and 755 underwent pulmonary angiography; 251 (33%) of 755 demonstrated pulmonary embolism. Almost all patients with pulmonary embolism had abnormal scans of high, intermediate, or low probability, but so did most without pulmonary embolism (sensitivity, 98%; specificity, 10%). Of 116 patients with high-probability scans and definitive angiograms, 102 (88%) had pulmonary embolism, but only a minority with pulmonary embolism had high-probability scans (sensitivity, 41%; specificity, 97%). Of 322 with intermediate-probability scans and definitive angiograms, 105 (33%) had pulmonary embolism. Follow-up and angiography together suggest pulmonary embolism occurred among 12% of patients with low-probability scans. Clinical assessment combined with the ventilation/perfusion scan established the diagnosis or exclusion of pulmonary embolism only for a minority of patients—those with clear and concordant clinical and ventilation/perfusion scan findings.

(*JAMA.* 1990;263:2753-2759)

PERFUSION lung scans have been reported to be sensitive in detecting pulmonary emboli, but many other conditions such as pneumonia or local bronchospasm cause perfusion defects.[1] Ventilation scans were added to perfusion scans with the idea that ventilation

For editorial comment see p 2794.

Reprint requests to Division of Lung Diseases, National Heart, Lung, and Blood Institute, Westwood Bldg, Room 6A16, 5333 Westbard Ave, Bethesda, MD 20892 (Carol E. Vreim, PhD).

would be abnormal in areas of pneumonia or local hypoventilation, but that in pulmonary embolism ventilation would be normal.[2] A number of investigators have attempted to make ventilation/perfusion (V̇/Q̇) scans more useful for diagnosing pulmonary embolism by classifying them not just as normal or abnormal, but if abnormal, as indicating high probability, intermediate probability (indeterminate), or low probability of pulmonary embolism.[3] Under the auspices of the National Heart, Lung, and Blood Institute, the Prospective Investigation of Pulmonary Embolism Diag-

nosis (PIOPED) investigators have assessed the diagnostic usefulness of V̇/Q̇ lung scans in acute pulmonary embolism. The project protocol and consent forms were approved by the institutional review boards of all participating centers. (Participating centers and investigators are listed at the end of the article.)

METHODS
Patient Enrollment

From January 1985 through September 1986 in each of six clinical centers, all patients for whom a request for a V̇/Q̇ scan or a pulmonary angiogram was made were considered for study entry. The eligible study population consisted of patients, 18 years or older, inpatients and outpatients, in whom symptoms that suggested pulmonary embolism were present within 24 hours of study entry and without contraindications to angiography such as pregnancy, serum creatinine level greater than 260 μmol/L, or hypersensitivity to contrast material. Once approached for the study, patients with recurrences were not approached for recruitment a second time.

Recruitment

A total of 5587 requests for V̇/Q̇ scans were recorded in the six PIOPED clinical centers from January 1985 through September 1986 (Figure). Although

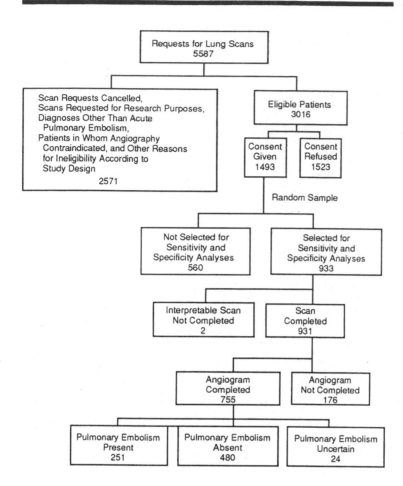

Flow chart illustrating the numbers of requests for lung scans, recruitment of patients, completion of lung scans, and results of angiography in the Prospective Investigation of Pulmonary Embolism Diagnosis.

some patients could not be thoroughly evaluated prior to completion of the V/Q scan, clinical investigators made every effort to record their individual clinical impressions as to the likelihood of pulmonary embolism prior to learning the results of V/Q scans and angiography. Impressions were based on an agreed on set of information—history, results of physical examination, arterial blood gas analyses, chest roentgenograms, and electrocardiograms—but without standardized diagnostic algorithms. The medical records of a random sample of patients who refused or were ineligible for study entry (refuser/ineligible patients) were evaluated retrospectively for comparison with study patients.

Lung Scan

The protocol directed ventilation and perfusion studies with the subject in the upright position, but other positions were acceptable. Ventilation studies were performed with 5.6×10^8 to 11.1×10^8 Bq of xenon 133 using a 20% symmetric window set over the 80-keV energy peak. They started with a 100 000-count, posterior-view, first-breath image and then posterior equilibrium (wash-in) images for two consecutive 120-second periods. Washout consisted of three serial 45-second posterior views, 45-second left and right posterior oblique views, and a final 45-second posterior view. Then, perfusion

scans were obtained with 1.5×10^8 Bq of technetium Tc 99m macroaggregated albumin that contained 100 000 to 700 000 particles using a 20% symmetric window set over the 140-keV energy peak. Particles were injected into an antecubital vein over 5 to 10 respiratory cycles, with the patient supine or at most semierect. The perfusion images consisted of anterior, posterior, both posterior oblique, and both anterior oblique views, with 750 000 counts per image for each. For the lateral view with the best perfusion, 500 000 counts per image were collected; the other lateral view was obtained for the same length of time. Scintillation cameras with a wide field of view (38.1 cm in diameter) were used with parallel-hole, low-energy, all-purpose collimators. Perfusion scans were satisfactory or better in 96% of cases, ventilation scans adequate or better in 95%.

Angiography

The femoral-vein Seldinger technique with a multiple side-holed, 6F to 8F pigtail catheter was used. Small amounts of contrast material (5 to 8 mL) were injected by hand, to check the patency of the inferior vena cava by fluoroscopy. The catheter was directed into the main pulmonary artery of the lung with the greatest V/Q scan abnormality. Initial filming was in the anteroposterior projection. Seventy-six percent iodinated contrast material was injected at a rate of 20 to 35 mL/s for a total of 40 to 50 mL (2-second injection). Film rates were three per second for 3 seconds, followed by one per second for 4 to 6 seconds. Depending on the size of the lungs, filming was not magnified or given a low magnification of 1.4. A 12:1 grid was used and roentgenographic factors were in the range of 70 to 80 kilovolts (peak) and 0.025 to 0.040 seconds at 1000 mA (large focal spot of 1.2 to 1.5 mm in diameter). If emboli were not identified, injections were repeated and magnification (1.8 to 2.0 times) oblique views were obtained of the areas suspicious for pulmonary embolism. Films were obtained with an air-gap technique (ie, no grid used). Roentgenographic factors were in the range of 78 to 88 kV(p) and 0.040 to 0.080 seconds at 160 mA (small focal spot of 0.3 to 0.6 mm in diameter). If no emboli were found in the first lung, or if bilateral angiography in the clinical center was routine, identical techniques were used for the second lung. Angiography was completed within 24 hours, and usually within 12 hours of V/Q scans. Pulmonary angiograms were adequate or better in 95% of cases.

Central Scan and Angiogram Interpretations

Two nuclear medicine readers, not from the center that performed the scan, independently interpreted the lung scans with chest roentgenograms according to preestablished study criteria (Table 1). Angiograms were likewise randomly assigned to pairs of angiographers from clinical centers other than the originating hospital. The angiogram readers interpreted the angiograms with lung scans as having acute pulmonary embolism present—which required the identification of an embolus obstructing a vessel or the outline of an embolus (filling defect) within a vessel—absent, or uncertain. If two readers disagreed, the interpretations were adjudicated by readers who were selected randomly from the remaining clinical centers. If adjudicating readers did not agree with either of the first two readers, scans or angiograms went to panels of nuclear medicine or angiography readers. The final adjudicated V/Q scan readings consisted of four categories—high probability, intermediate probability (indeterminate), low probability, and low/very low probability through normal (near normal/normal). The near-normal/normal category includes readings of very low probability by one reader and low probability by the other, very low probability by both, very low probability by one and normal by the other, and normal by both. Refuser/ineligible patients' scans were read in each clinical center by the clinical center's PIOPED nuclear medicine reader(s) and not reread.

Follow-up and Outcome Classification

Patients were contacted by telephone at 1, 3, 6, and 12 months after study entry. Deaths, new studies for pulmonary embolism, and major bleeding complications were reviewed by an outcome classification committee using all available information. Only 23 (2.5%) of the 931 patients had incomplete (16) or no (7) follow-up. Angiograms, follow-up data, and outcome classifications were used to determine pulmonary embolism status as positive for patients with angiograms that showed pulmonary emboli and for patients for whom outcome review established the presence of pulmonary emboli at the time of PIOPED recruitment. Pulmonary embolism status was determined as negative for patients with angiograms that did not show pulmonary emboli and no contrary outcome review and for patients who lacked a definitive angiogram reading who were discharged from the hospital without a prescription for anticoagu-

Table 1.—PIOPED Central Scan Interpretation Categories and Criteria*

High probability
≥2 Large (>75% of a segment) segmental perfusion defects without corresponding ventilation or roentgenographic abnormalities or substantially larger than either matching ventilation or chest roentgenogram abnormalities
≥2 Moderate segmental (≥25% and ≤75% of a segment) perfusion defects without matching ventilation or chest roentgenogram abnormalities and 1 large mismatched segmental defect
≥4 Moderate segmental perfusion defects without ventilation or chest roentgenogram abnormalities

Intermediate probability (indeterminate)
Not falling into normal, very-low-, low-, or high-probability categories
Borderline high or borderline low
Difficult to categorize as low or high

Low probability
Nonsegmental perfusion defects (eg, very small effusion causing blunting of the costophrenic angle, cardiomegaly, enlarged aorta, hila, and mediastinum, and elevated diaphragm)
Single moderate mismatched segmental perfusion defect with normal chest roentgenogram
Any perfusion defect with a substantially *larger* chest roentgenogram abnormality
Large or moderate segmental perfusion defects involving no more than 4 segments in 1 lung and no more than 3 segments in 1 lung region with *matching* ventilation defects either equal to or larger in size and chest roentgenogram either normal or with abnormalities substantially smaller than perfusion defects
>3 Small segmental perfusion defects (<25% of a segment) with a normal chest roentgenogram

Very low probability
≤3 Small segmental perfusion defects with a normal chest roentgenogram

Normal
No perfusion defects present
Perfusion outlines exactly the shape of the lungs as seen on the chest roentgenogram (hilar and aortic impressions may be seen, chest roentgenogram and/or ventilation study may be abnormal)

*PIOPED indicates Prospective Investigation of Pulmonary Embolism Diagnosis.

Table 2.—Recruitment of Patients and Completion of Angiography*

Clinical Center	% of Eligible Patients Recruited	No. of PIOPED Patients With Lung Scans Who Were Selected for Angiographic Pursuit	Angiograms Obtained, No. (%)
Duke University	46	137	115 (84)
Henry Ford Hospital	62	228	177 (78)
Massachusetts General Hospital	33	140	120 (86)
University of Michigan	52	102	65 (64)
University of Pennsylvania	70	168	134 (80)
Yale University	43	156	144 (92)
Total	50	931	755 (81)

*PIOPED indicates Prospective Investigation of Pulmonary Embolism Diagnosis.

lants and in whom no outcome event suggested pulmonary embolism. Pulmonary embolism status could be determined as positive or negative for 902 patients. A clinical assessment of the likelihood of pulmonary embolism was available for 887 (98%) of these patients.

Statistical Methods

Probability values for the comparison of percentages and proportions and 95% confidence intervals (CIs) were calculated using standard z tests.[4] A χ^2 test for homogeneity of proportions was used to compare distributions.[5] *Sensitivity* is defined as the proportion of cases of pulmonary embolism correctly diagnosed and *specificity* as the proportion of diagnoses that pulmonary embolism is absent for patients without pulmonary embolism. Sensitivity, specificity, and percent agreement have been calculated according to standard methods for proportions.[6] Analyses were performed with the Statistical Package for the Social Sciences statistical software package.[7] Recruitment of

900 to 1000 patients in the random sample for PIOPED angiography was planned to obtain estimates of sensitivity and specificity with 95% CIs no wider than ±8%. To determine the sensitivity and specificity of V/Q lung scans without the biases associated with haphazard patient selection (ie, convenience sampling),[8,9] a 933-patient sample of the 1493 patients who consented to PIOPED participation was selected according to random sampling schedules created separately by the data and coordinating center for each clinical center. The PIOPED protocol required these 933 patients to undergo angiography if their scans were abnormal. Of the 933 patients selected for angiography, 1 patient died before the V/Q scan could be completed and 1 other patient's V/Q scan was determined to be uninterpretable. These 2 patients are not further reported herein.

RESULTS

Of the 3016 patients eligible for PIOPED, 1493 (50%) gave consent to

Table 3.—Patient Characteristics*

	PIOPED (N=931)	Refuser/ Ineligible (N=326)
Age (mean), y	56.1	56.4
Male, %	45	44
Service, %		
Medical/CCU	40	36
Surgical	18	21
Emergency department/clinic	30	32
ICU	10	10
Other	1	1
Hospital mortality, %	9	10

*PIOPED indicates Prospective Investigation of Pulmonary Embolism Diagnosis; CCU, coronary care unit; and ICU, intensive care unit.

Table 4.—Comparison of Scan Category With Angiogram Findings

Scan Category	Pulmonary Embolism Present	Pulmonary Embolism Absent	Pulmonary Embolism Uncertain	No Angiogram	Total No.
High probability	102	14	1	7	124
Intermediate probability	105	217	9	33	364
Low probability	39	199	12	62	312
Near normal/normal	5	50	2	74	131
Total	251	480	24	176	931

Table 5.—Comparison of Scan Category With Angiogram Findings, Sensitivity and Specificity

Scan Category	Sensitivity, %	Specificity, %
High probability	41	97
High or intermediate probability	82	52
High, intermediate, or low probability	98	10

participate in PIOPED (Figure). The clinical centers varied in the percentage of eligible patients for whom consent could be obtained, from 33% to 70%, and in the percentage of patients for whom angiograms were obtained among those selected to determine the sensitivity and specificity of V/Q lung scans (PIOPED angiographic pursuit), from 64% to 92% (Table 2). The PIOPED patients resembled refuser/ineligible patients in a variety of clinical characteristics (Table 3). The PIOPED patients and refuser/ineligible patients were different, however, in their lung scan abnormalities ($P<.01$). Although they had similar frequencies of high-probability scans (13% among PIOPED patients and 11% among refuser/ineligible patients), the PIOPED patients had intermediate-probability scans almost twice as often as refuser/ineligible patients (39% vs 22%). The PIOPED study had a smaller proportion of patients with low-probability and near-normal/normal lung scans. Of the 931 patients who were selected for mandatory angiography in PIOPED, 755 (81.1%) completed angiography; 69 (7.4%) did not complete angiography because their V/Q scans were interpreted locally as normal; and 107 (11.5%) did not complete angiography in spite of the requirements of the protocol.

Reader Agreement

Agreement among scan readers was excellent for high-probability (95%), very-low-probability (92%), and normal (94%) scan categories. For intermediate-probability (indeterminate) and low-probability scan categories, the readers agreed less frequently (75% and 70%, respectively). In only 24 (2.6%) of 931 scans was panel adjudication necessary. Agreement among angiogram readers was excellent for the presence of pulmonary embolism (92%). For the absence of pulmonary embolism and pulmonary embolism uncertain, independent readers agreed on 83% and 89%

of angiograms, respectively. In only 13 (1.7%) of 755 angiograms was panel adjudication necessary.

Scan Findings

Most (676) of the 931 patients had intermediate- or low-probability V/Q scan readings (39% and 34%, respectively) (Table 4). Only 131 (14%) had near-normal/normal V/Q scans and 124 (13%) had high-probability scans. The 176 patients who did not undergo angiography, in spite of their selection for mandatory angiography, had less severe scan abnormalities than those who completed angiography ($P<.01$).

Angiogram and Outcome Findings

Among the 755 patients who completed angiography, 251 (33%) had thromboemboli seen on the angiogram, 480 (64%) had no thromboemboli seen, and 24 (3%) had angiograms in which the presence of thromboemboli was uncertain (Table 4). For the vast majority of patients, 1 year of follow-up revealed clinical courses entirely consistent with angiographically established diagnoses. The outcome classification committee disagreed with central angiography interpretations for 4 patients with pulmonary angiograms free of signs of acute embolism who had pulmonary embolism at autopsies performed 2 to 6 days after angiography. The scan interpretations were of low probability for 3 and of intermediate probability (indeterminate) for 1 of these 4 patients.

Scans Compared With Angiograms

One hundred two of 251 patients with angiograms that showed thromboemboli had high-probability V/Q scans. The sensitivity, therefore, was 41% (95% CI, 34% to 47%) (Tables 4 and 5). If the patient had either a high- or intermediate-probability V/Q scan, the sen-

sitivity for thromboemboli on angiography increased to 207 (82%) of 251 (95% CI, 78% to 87%). If the patient had either a high-, intermediate-, or low-probability V/Q scan, then 246 of 251 had thromboemboli on angiography, a sensitivity of 98% (95% CI, 96% to 100%).

Only 14 (3%) of 480 patients who did not have thromboemboli on angiography had high-probability V/Q scans. The specificity of a high-probability scan—ie, the percentage of patients with angiograms free of signs of acute embolism who had a scan that showed other than high probability—was 97% (466/480) (95% CI, 96% to 98%). For high- and intermediate-probability scans together, specificity was 52% (249/480 patients with angiograms free of signs of acute embolism) (95% CI, 47% to 56%). For high-, intermediate-, and low-probability scans together, specificity was 10% (50/480 patients with angiograms free of signs of acute embolism) (95% CI, 8% to 13%). The 36 sensitivities and specificities calculated by reproducing Table 5 for each clinical center varied about the studywide sensitivities and specificities—25 (69%) of 36 were within ±5% of the studywide estimates and 34 (94%) of 36 within ±10%.

Most patients with high-probability V/Q scans had angiographic evidence of pulmonary embolism (102/116 definitive studies, or a positive predictive value of 88%). Of the 60 patients with previous histories of pulmonary embolism, 20 were found to have pulmonary emboli on angiography. Of the 19 patients with histories of pulmonary embolism and a high-probability V/Q scan, only 14 were found to have acute pulmonary emboli on angiography. The positive predictive value of a high-probability V/Q scan in patients with histories of pulmonary

Ventilation/Perfusion Scan—PIOPED Investigators

Session 2 – Diagnosis & asking answerable clinical questions

Table 6.—Pulmonary Embolism (PE) Status*

Scan Category	Clinical Science Probability, %							
	80-100		20-79		0-19		All Probabilities	
	PE + /No. of Patients	%	PE + /No. of Patients	%	PE + /No. of Patients	%	PE + /No. of Patients	%
High probability	28/29	96	70/80	88	5/9	56	103/118	87
Intermediate probability	27/41	66	66/236	28	11/68	16	104/345	30
Low probability	6/15	40	30/191	16	4/90	4	40/296	14
Near normal/normal	0/5	0	4/62	6	1/61	2	5/128	4
Total	61/90	68	170/569	30	21/228	9	252/887	28

*PE + indicates angiogram reading that shows pulmonary embolism or determination of pulmonary embolism by the outcome classification committee on review. Pulmonary embolism status is based on angiogram interpretation for 713 patients, on angiogram interpretation and outcome classification committee reassignment for 4 patients, and on clinical information alone (without definitive angiography) for 170 patients.

embolism was only 74% (14/19), compared with 91% (88/97) for those without a history of pulmonary embolism ($P<.05$). This difference in positive predictive values reflects a loss of specificity in the high-probability V/Q scan diagnosis for patients with histories of pulmonary embolism (88%) vs those with no prior pulmonary embolism (98%) ($P<.01$).

The percentage of patients whose angiograms showed thromboemboli was less in the intermediate-probability (indeterminate), low-probability, and near-normal/normal scan categories— 33%, 16%, and 9%, respectively (Table 4). The frequency of angiographically demonstrable emboli among patients with low-probability scans (39 [16%] of 238) and near-normal/normal scans (5 [9%] of 55) is influenced by the relatively large numbers of patients (74 patients and 76 patients, respectively) for whom angiography was not completed or interpretations were uncertain in these scan categories (Table 4). Since none of these patients received anticoagulants and none developed clinically evident pulmonary embolism during follow-up, important pulmonary emboli did not occur in this group. If all 150 patients were regarded as not having had pulmonary emboli, then the frequency of clinically important pulmonary emboli in patients with low-probability scans could be no less than 39 (12%) of 312, and in patients with near-normal/normal scans, 5 (4%) of 131.

There were 21 patients whose V/Q scans were read centrally as normal on first reading by both readers. Three underwent angiography and none showed thromboemboli. None of the remaining 18 patients received anticoagulants and none had clinically evident pulmonary embolism on follow-up.

Clinical Assessment of the Likelihood of Pulmonary Embolism

The clinician's assessment of the likelihood of pulmonary embolism recorded before the scan was performed ("prior probability") was compared with pulmonary embolism status as determined by angiography and follow-up information (Table 6) for 887 patients with prior probability assessments and definite pulmonary embolism status. A clinical assessment of 80% to 100% likelihood of pulmonary embolism was made in 90 patients (10%) and was correct in 61 (68%) of 90. A clinical assessment of 0% to 19% likelihood of pulmonary embolism was made in 228 (26%) and was correct in 207 (91%) of 228. Clinical assessment, therefore, was more often correct in excluding pulmonary embolism than in identifying pulmonary embolism. In the majority of patients (569 [64%]), clinical assessments were noncommittal (20% to 79% likelihood of pulmonary embolism).

Combining clinical assessments with the V/Q scan interpretations improved the overall chance of reaching a correct diagnosis of acute pulmonary embolism (Table 6). Among patients in whom the clinical impression and the scan interpretation were both of high probability for pulmonary embolism, 28 (96%) of 29 had pulmonary embolism. If the high-probability scan interpretation was paired with an intermediate-likelihood clinical assessment or a low-likelihood clinical assessment, then the probability that the patient had pulmonary embolism fell to 70 (88%) of 80 and 5 (56%) of 9, respectively. The addition of the clinical evaluation also helped in the low-probability and in the near-normal/normal scan categories. A low-probability clinical assessment (0% to 19% likelihood of pulmonary embolism based on clinical judgment), when paired with a low-probability V/Q scan, correctly excluded the diagnosis of pulmonary embolism in 86 (96%) of 90 patients. The near-normal/normal V/Q scan category, when paired with a low-likelihood clinical assessment, correctly excluded pulmonary embolism in 60 (98%) of 61 patients.

COMMENT

The PIOPED study was conducted as a multicenter, prospective effort to estimate the sensitivity and specificity of the V/Q lung scan for the diagnosis of pulmonary embolism. Other retrospective and prospective studies have focused on positive predictive values, which are influenced by prevalence of pulmonary embolism and patient selection. Sensitivity and specificity, however, are fundamental characteristics of a diagnostic test and are not affected by the prevalence of disease.[10]

In PIOPED, almost all patients (98%) with clinically important pulmonary embolism had lung scans that fell into one of the three abnormal categories— high, intermediate (indeterminate), or low probability. If all three abnormal categories are combined into one, the lung scan is sensitive enough to serve as a screening test for the diagnosis of pulmonary embolism, but the specificity is limited. The high-probability scan lacked sensitivity in diagnosing pulmonary embolism, since it failed to identify 59% of patients with this disorder.

Only 14 (3%) of 480 patients who did not have evidence of acute pulmonary embolism on angiography had high-probability scans (Table 4). Therefore, the specificity of a high-probability scan was 97%. For patients with histories of pulmonary embolism, the specificity of the high-probability scan was reduced. This finding is consistent with other reports of previous pulmonary embolism as a cause of V/Q scan abnormality that may be confused with acute pulmonary embolism.[11,12] The specificity of scans of intermediate or low probability was much less than the specificity of the high-probability scan.

The PIOPED's study design included patient enumeration and recruitment prior to scan completion to avoid bias in patient selection. Nonetheless, patients who ultimately had high- and intermediate-probability scans were more often successfully recruited for PIOPED. If anything, this selection bias would suggest that PIOPED tends to overestimate V/Q scans' sensitivities and underestimate specificities.

Clinical decisions are often made on the basis of the predictive values, which depend not only on the test's sensitivity and specificity, but also on the prevalence of disease in the population studied. Based on angiogram results, the prevalence of pulmonary embolism in PIOPED was 33% (251/755) (Table 4); based on pulmonary embolism status—derived from angiogram evaluation and/or clinical evaluation—the prevalence was 28% (Table 6), similar to the prevalences described in previous reports.[13-21] In PIOPED, the positive predictive value of the high-probability scan was 88%, whereas the negative predictive value of a low-probability scan was 84%. The negative predictive value of the near-normal/normal scan category was better at 91%. Estimates of negative predictive values increased when analyses took into account patients who did not undergo angiography, did not receive anticoagulants, and had no evidence of pulmonary embolism occurring during 1 year of follow-up. Including these patients among those not having pulmonary embolism in the analysis improved the negative predictive value of the low-probability scan from 84% to 88% and of the near-normal/normal scan from 91% to 96%. Because some instances of acute pulmonary embolism may not have been detected among these patients, the true negative predictive values may be less than 88% for low-probability scans and 96% for near-normal/normal scans, but still ought to be closer to these latter values than to the 84% and 91%, which did not account for patients without angiography results.

Although pulmonary emboli did occur in patients with scans classified in the categories between low probability and normal, pulmonary embolism was documented in only 5 (4%) of 131 of such patients. The true proportion of patients with pulmonary embolism must be inferred with caution, because large numbers of patients with near-normal/normal scans were not successfully recruited for the study. Only 42% of the 131 PIOPED patients in this category completed angiography. Only 3 of the 21 patients with lung scans read as normal by both readers on the final reading completed angiography; all 3 had normal pulmonary angiograms. None of the remaining 18 had clinically evident pulmonary emboli on follow-up. This finding is consistent with the findings of Kipper et al.[22]

The value of combining clinical judgment with the interpretation of the scan is supported by the PIOPED study. The predictive value of the high- and low-probability lung scans improved when supported by similar clinical assessments. For 90 patients, the negative predictive value of the low-probability scan rose to 96% when accompanied by a clinical assessment of low likelihood. In 29 patients, the positive predictive value of a high-probability scan increased to 96% if supported by a high-likelihood clinical assessment. In the PIOPED experience, combining a lung scan interpretation with a strong clinical suspicion as to whether acute pulmonary embolism is present is a sound diagnostic strategy, as previously suggested by McNeil and colleagues,[20,21] but is sufficient for only a minority of patients (Table 6). For a substantial number of patients in the PIOPED study, angiography was required for a definitive diagnosis of pulmonary embolism.

The PIOPED study employed pulmonary angiography, which proved to be a safe and accurate method of diagnosing pulmonary embolism, although it is invasive. The four patients (0.5%) for whom the outcome classification committee disagreed with blinded angiogram interpretations that showed acute pulmonary embolism to be absent must be considered carefully in light of the angiographic criteria's design for acute pulmonary embolism, the variable time between angiographic evaluation and the patients' deaths, and the variability in pathophysiology and pathological interpretation of thromboemboli in evolution. In the PIOPED study, a normal angiogram almost excluded the possibility of pulmonary embolism, confirming the results of two previous studies.[14,15]

The PIOPED findings extend observations made by other investigators,[1-3,12-20] from whom the PIOPED investigators derived study criteria for angiogram and V/Q scan interpretation. Although predictive values for patients with high-probability scans and patients with low-probability scans in previous series are generally consistent with the PIOPED findings, the underrepresentation of patients with low-probability scans in previous studies has in the past led to an exaggerated impression of the sensitivity of the high-probability lung scan.

The findings of Hull and colleagues[17,18] in the Hamilton District Thromboembolism Programme are particularly interesting in comparison with the PIOPED results. Of the 305 patients with suspected pulmonary embolism and abnormal perfusion lung scans in their study, 173 (57%) had adequate ventilation scans and adequate pulmonary angio-

grams. Ninety-five patients (31%) had pulmonary emboli demonstrated on angiography. The predictive values from their study are similar to PIOPED results in the high-probability and intermediate-probability (indeterminate) scan categories. The PIOPED study, likewise, found pulmonary emboli among patients with scans in the low-probability category, but fewer than the 25% for subsegmental matched lesions and 40% for subsegmental mismatched lesions found by Hull et al. Patient referral patterns or lung scan interpretation criteria may account for the differences between PIOPED results and the Hamilton study results. Since angiographic studies are not available and clinical follow-up has not been applied to determine pulmonary embolism status for the 110 patients without adequate angiography, for the 22 patients without adequate ventilation scans, and for the patients with normal scans in the Hamilton District Thromboembolism Programme, comparisons of estimates of sensitivity and specificity between the two studies are not possible.

The PIOPED results lead to a number of conclusions that settle controversies about the diagnostic value of the lung scan in pulmonary embolism.[23,24] A high-probability scan usually indicates pulmonary embolism, but only a minority of patients with pulmonary embolism have a high-probability scan. A history of pulmonary embolism decreases the accuracy of diagnoses based on high-probability scans. A low-probability scan with a strong clinical impression that pulmonary embolism is not likely makes the possibility of pulmonary embolism remote. Near-normal/normal lung scans make the diagnosis of acute pulmonary embolism very unlikely. An intermediate-probability (indeterminate) scan is not of help in establishing a diagnosis. In PIOPED, the scan combined with clinical assessment permitted a noninvasive diagnosis or exclusion of acute pulmonary embolism for a minority of patients.

This study was supported by contracts N01-HR-34007, N01-HR-34008, N01-HR-34009, N01-HR-34010, N01-HR-34011, N01-HR-34012, and N01-HR-34013 from the National Heart, Lung, and Blood Institute, Bethesda, Md.

The secretarial assistance of JoAnne Decker has been greatly appreciated.

Steering Committee

The PIOPED investigators are as follows:

Herbert A. Saltzman, MD, chairman; Abass Alavi, MD, Richard H. Greenspan, MD, Charles A. Hales, MD, Paul D. Stein, MD, Michael Terrin, MD, MPH, Carol Vreim, PhD, John G. Weg, MD; alternates: Christos Athanasoulis, MD, Alexander Gottschalk, MD.

Session 2 – Diagnosis & asking answerable clinical questions

Clinical Centers

Duke University
Herbert A. Saltzman, MD, principal investigator; Russell Blinder, MD, R. Edward Coleman, MD, N. Reed Dunnick, MD, William J. Fulkerson, Jr, MD, Lee Mallatratt, RN, Carl E. Ravin, MD.

Henry Ford Hospital
Paul D. Stein, MD, principal investigator; Deborah Adams, RN, Matthew Burke, MD, Jerry W. Froelich, MD, Kenneth V. Leeper, MD, Barry A. Lesser, MD, John Popovich, Jr, MD, P. C. Shetty, MD, James Thrall, MD.

Massachusetts General Hospital
Charles A. Hales, MD, principal investigator; Christos Athanasoulis, MD, Stuart Geller, MD, Kenneth McKusick, MD, Deborah Quinn, RN, MS, B. Taylor Thompson, MD, Arthur C. Waltman, MD.

University of Michigan
John G. Weg, MD, principal investigator; Grace Ball, RN, Kyung J. Cho, MD, Charles A. Easton, MD, Andrew Flint, MD, Thomas A. Griggs, MD, Jack E. Juni, MD, Jerold Wallis, MD, David Williams, MD.

University of Pennsylvania
Abass Alavi, MD, principal investigator; Margaret Ahearn-Spera, RNC, MSN, Dana R. Burke, MD, Jeffrey Carson, MD, Mark A. Kelley, MD, Gordon K. McLean, MD, Steven G. Meranze, MD, Harold I. Palevsky, MD, Sanford Schwartz, MD.

Yale University
Richard H. Greenspan, MD, principal investigator; Donald F. Denny, Jr, MD, Alexander Gottschalk, MD, Lee H. Greenwood, MD, Jacob S. O. Loke, MD, Richard A. Matthay, MD, Steven S. Morse, MD, H. Dirk Sostman, MD, Felicia Tencza, MPH.

Data and Coordinating Center

Maryland Medical Research Institute: Michael L. Terrin, MD, MPH, principal investigator; Wilmot Ball, MD, Mary Burke, Martha Canner, MS, Paul Canner, PhD, Margie Carroll, Martin Goldman, MD, Carol Handy, Elizabeth Heinz, Thomas E. Hobbins, MD, Frank Hooper, ScD, Steven Kaufman, MD, Christian R. Klimt, MD, DrPH (principal investigator, September 1983 through September 1984), William F. Krol, PhD, Norman LaFrance, MD, Gerard J. Prud'homme, MA, Sharon Pruitt, Pauline Raiz, Bruce Thompson, PhD, Heidi Weissman, MD.

Project Office

National Heart, Lung, and Blood Institute: Carol E. Vreim, PhD, Margaret Wu, PhD.

Policy and Data Safety Monitoring Board

Myron Stein, MD, chairman; Daniel M. Biello, MD (deceased), Sarah Greene Burger, MPH, Robert Henkin, MD, Thomas Hyers, MD, Paul S. Levy, ScD, Franklin Miller, Jr, MD, Robert E. O'Mara, MD, Morris Simon, MD, Gerard Turino, MD, George W. Williams, PhD.

Outcome Classification Committee

Mark A. Kelley, MD, chairman; Jeffrey Carson, MD, William J. Fulkerson, MD, Thomas E. Hobbins, MD, Richard A. Matthay, MD, Harold Palevsky, MD, John Popovich, Jr, MD, B. Taylor Thompson, MD, John G. Weg, MD.

References

1. Wagner HN, Sabiston DC, Iio M, McAfee JG, Meyer JK, Langan JK. Regional pulmonary blood flow in man by radioisotope scanning. *JAMA.* 1964;187:601-603.
2. Wagner HN Jr, Lopez-Majano V, Langan JK, Joshi RC. Radioactive xenon in the differential diagnosis of pulmonary embolism. *Radiology.* 1968;91:1168-1184.
3. Biello DR, Mattar AG, McKnight RC, Siegel BA. Ventilation perfusion studies in suspected pulmonary embolism. *Am J Radiol.* 1979;133:1033-1037.
4. Snedecor JW, Cochran WG. *Statistical Methods.* 6th ed. Ames: Iowa State University Press; 1967.
5. Cochran WG. Some methods of strengthening the common χ^2 tests. *Biometrics.* 1954;10:417-451.
6. Fleiss JL. *Statistical Methods for Rates and Proportions.* 2nd ed. New York, NY: John Wiley & Sons Inc; 1981.
7. Nie NH, ed. *SPSS^x User's Guide.* New York, NY: McGraw-Hill International Book Co; 1983.
8. Hill AB. *Principles of Medical Statistics.* 9th ed. New York, NY: Oxford University Press Inc; 1971.
9. Murphy EA. *Probability in Medicine.* Baltimore, Md: The Johns Hopkins University Press; 1979.
10. Vecchio JJ. Predictive value of a single diagnostic test in unselected populations. *N Engl J Med.* 1966;274:1171-1175.
11. Li DK, Seltzer SG, McNeil BJ. V/Q mismatches unassociated with pulmonary embolism: case report and review of the literature. *J Nucl Med.* 1978;19:1331-1333.
12. Biello DR, Kumar B. Symmetrical perfusion defects without pulmonary embolism. *Eur J Nucl Med.* 1982;7:197-199.
13. Alderson PO, Martin EC. Pulmonary embolism: diagnosis with multiple imaging modalities. *Radiology.* 1987;164:297-312.
14. Cheely R, McCartney WH, Perry JR, et al. The role of noninvasive tests versus pulmonary angiography in the diagnosis of pulmonary embolism. *Am J Med.* 1981;70:17-22.
15. Novelline RA, Baitarowich OH, Athanasoulis CA, Waltman AC, Greenfield AJ, Mckusick KA. The clinical course of patients with suspected pulmonary embolism and a negative pulmonary arteriogram. *Radiology.* 1978;126:561-567.
16. Sasahara AA, Stein M, Simon M, Littmann D. Pulmonary angiography in the diagnosis of thromboembolic disease. *N Engl J Med.* 1964;270:1075-1081.
17. Hull RD, Hirsh J, Carter CJ, et al. Pulmonary angiography, ventilation lung scanning and venography for clinically suspected pulmonary embolism with abnormal perfusion lung scan. *Ann Intern Med.* 1983;98:891-899.
18. Hull RD, Hirsh J, Carter CJ, et al. Diagnostic value of ventilation-perfusion lung scanning in patients with suspected pulmonary embolism. *Chest.* 1985;88:819-828.
19. Poulose KP, Reba RC, Gilday DL, Deland FH, Wagner HN. Diagnosis of pulmonary embolism: a correlative study of the clinical, scan, and angiographic findings. *BMJ.* 1970;3:67-71.
20. McNeil BJ. Ventilation-perfusion studies and the diagnoses of pulmonary embolism: concise communication. *J Nucl Med.* 1980;21:319-323.
21. McNeil BJ, Hessel SJ, Branch WT, Bjork L, Adelstein SJ. Measures of clinical efficacy, III: the value of the lung scan in the evaluation of young patients with pleuritic chest pain. *J Nucl Med.* 1976;17:163-169.
22. Kipper MS, Moser KM, Kortman KE, Ashburn WL. Long-term follow-up of patients with suspected pulmonary embolism and a normal lung scan. *Chest.* 1982;82:411-415.
23. Robin ED. Over diagnosis and over treatment of pulmonary embolism: the emperor may have no clothes. *Ann Intern Med.* 1977;87:775-781.
24. Biello DR. Radiological (scintigraphic) evaluation of patients with suspected pulmonary thromboembolism. *JAMA.* 1987;257:3257-3259.

Citation:

Are the results of this diagnostic study valid?

Was there an independent, blind comparison with
a reference ('gold') standard of diagnosis?

Was the diagnostic test evaluated in an appropriate
spectrum of patients (like those in whom it would
be used in practice)?

Was the reference standard applied regardless of
the diagnostic test result?

Are the valid results of this diagnostic study important?

SAMPLE CALCULATIONS (see p120 of *Evidence-based Medicine*)

		Target disorder (iron deficiency anaemia)		Totals
		Present	Absent	
Diagnostic test result	Positive (<65 mmol/L)	731 a	270 b	a+b 1001
(serum ferritin)	Negative (≥65 mmol/L)	78 c	1500 d	c+d 1578
	Totals	809 a+c	1770 b+d	a+b+c+d 2579

Sensitivity = a/(a+c) = 731/809 = 90%

Specificity = d/(b+d) = 1500/1770 = 85%

Likelihood Ratio for a positive test result = LR+=sens/(1-spec)=90%/15%=6

Likelihood Ratio for a negative test result=LR-=(1-sens)/spec=10%/85%=0.12

Positive Predictive Value = a/(a+b) = 731/1001 = 73%

Negative Predictive Value = d/(c+d) = 1500/1578 = 95%

Pre-test Probability (prevalence) = (a+c)/(a+b+c+d) = 809/2579 = 32%

Pre-test-odds = prevalence/(1-prevalence) = 31%/69% = 0.45

Post-test odds = Pre-test odds x Likelihood Ratio

Post-test Probability = Post-test odds/(Post-test odds + 1)

Are the valid results of this diagnostic study important?

YOUR CALCULATIONS

		Target disorder		Totals
		Present	**Absent**	
Diagnostic test result	Positive	a	b	a+b
	Negative	c	d	c+d
	Totals	a+c	b+d	a+b+c+d

Sensitivity = a/(a+c) =   Specificity = d/(b+d) =

Likelihood Ratio for a positive test result = LR+=sens/(1-spec)=

Likelihood Ratio for a negative test result=LR-=(1-sens)/spec=

Positive Predictive Value = a/(a+b) =   Negative Predictive Value = d/(c+d) =

Pre-test Probability (prevalence) = (a+c)/(a+b+c+d) =

Pre-test-odds = prevalence/(1-prevalence) =

Post-test odds = Pre-test odds x Likelihood Ratio =

Post-test Probability = Post-test odds/(Post-test odds + 1) =

Can you apply this valid, important evidence about a diagnostic test in caring for your patient?

Is the diagnostic test available, affordable, accurate, and precise in your setting?

Can you generate a clinically sensible estimate of your patient's pre-test probability (from practice data, personal experience, the report itself, or clinical speculation)?

Will the resulting post-test probabilities affect your management and help your patient? (Could it move you across a test-treatment threshold? Would your patient be a willing partner in carrying it out?)

Would the consequences of the test help your patient?

Additional notes

A LIKELIHOOD RATIO NOMOGRAM

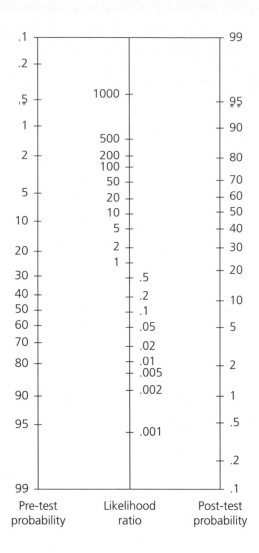

Anchor a straight-edge along the left edge of the nomogram at your patient's pre-test probability and pivot it until it intersects the likelihood ratio for your patient's diagnostic test result. It will intersect the right edge of the nomogram at your patient's post-test probability. Test 1: for a likelihood ratio of 1, pre-test and post-test probabilities should be identical. Test 2: for a pre-test probability of 30% and a likelihood ratio of 5, the post-test probability is just under 70%.

Adapted from Fagan TJ (1975) Nomogram for Bayes' theorem. *N Engl J Med.* **293**: 257.

Citation: The PIOPED investigators. Value of the ventilation/perfusion scan in acute pulmonary embolism. *JAMA* 1990; **263**: 2753-9

Are the results of this diagnostic study valid?

Was there an independent, blind comparison with a reference ('gold') standard of diagnosis?

Yes. Positive gold standard was pulmonary angiography. Negative gold standard was either angiography or benign clinical course or no treatment.

Was the diagnostic test evaluated in an appropriate spectrum of patients (like those in whom it would be used in practice)?

Yes.

Was the reference standard applied regardless of the diagnostic test result?

No – see No 1. Could not justify angiography in patients with normal lung scans.

Are the valid results of this diagnostic study important?

(*see* pp 122–128 of *Evidence-based Medicine*)

Lung scan result	Pulmonary embolism present	Pulmonary embolism absent[1]	Likelihood ratio
High probability	102/251 = 0.406	22/680 = 0.032	13
Intermediate probability	105/251 = 0.418	259/680 = 0.381	1.1
Low probability	39/251 = 0.155	273/680 = 0.401	0.38
Normal/near normal	5/251 = 0.020	126/680 = 0.185	0.11
Totals	251	680	

[1]150 patients with low probability or normal lung scans either didn't undergo angiography or their diagnosis of pulmonary embolism was uncertain; however, none were treated and all had a benign clinical course, so it appears safe to place them in the 'pulmonary embolism absent' column. The same appears to be the case for 50 patients with intermediate probability lung scans, so we have handled them in the same way.

Can you apply this valid, important evidence about a diagnostic test in caring for your patient?

Is the diagnostic test available, affordable, accurate, and precise in your setting?	**Needs to be assessed in each setting.**
Can you generate a clinically sensible estimate of your patient's pre-test probability (from practice data, personal experience, the report itself, or clinical speculation)?	**We reckoned it was about 50%.**
Will the resulting post-test probabilities affect your management and help your patient? (Could it move you across a test-treatment threshold? Would your patient be a willing partner in carrying it out?)	**With a high probability scan (LR 13), post test probability rose to 13/14 or 93%.**
Would the consequences of the test help your patient?	**Confirmed her diagnosis, and would strengthen our resolve to complete her treatment if she had a minor bleed in the second week of therapy.**

Additional notes

But what would you do if her lung scan had been reported as 'intermediate' probability? (Her pre-scan to post-scan probability of pulmonary embolism would only shift from 50% to 52%.)

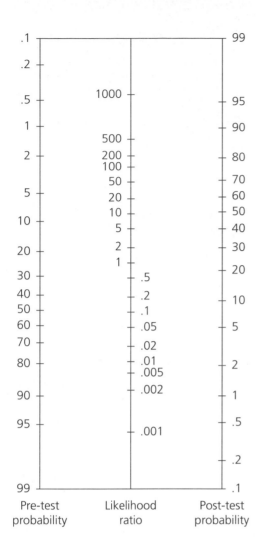

Anchor a straight-edge along the left edge of the nomogram at your patient's pre-test probability and pivot it until it intersects the likelihood ratio for your patient's diagnostic test result. It will intersect the right edge of the nomogram at your patient's post-test probability. Test 1: for a likelihood ratio of 1, pre-test and post-test probabilities should be identical. Test 2: for a pre-test probability of 30% and a likelihood ratio of 5, the post-test probability is just under 70%.

Adapted from Fagan TJ (1975) Nomogram for Bayes' theorem. *N Engl J Med.* **293**: 257.

PULMONARY EMBOLISM – VENTILATION/PERFUSION SCANS CAN BE DIAGNOSTIC IN ACUTE PULMONARY EMBOLISM (PIOPED)

Appraised by Sharon Straus Nov 1996.
Expiry date: 1998.

Clinical Bottom Line(s)

1 In a patient with suspected PE, a high probability V/Q scan virtually rules in PE, and a normal/near normal scan virtually rules it out.

2 An intermediate probability scan does not shift the probability of PE, and further testing should be done.

Citation

The PIOPED investigators. Value of the ventilation/perfusion scan in acute pulmonary embolism. *JAMA* 1990; **263:** 2753–9.

Clinical Question

In patients with clinically suspected pulmonary embolism, how sensitive and specific is a 'high-probability' V/Q scan?

Search Terms

'pulmonary embolism', 'lung scan' in MEDLINE

The Study

1 Gold Standard – pulmonary angio or clinical follow-up

2 Study Setting – prospective study of pts referred for V/Q scan at 6 clinical centres in the US

The Evidence

Test result	PE present	PE absent	LR
High probability scan	102/251 = 0.406	*22/680 = 0.032	13
Intermediate probability scan	105/251 = 0.418	*259/680 = 0.381	1.1
Low probability scan	39/251 = 0.155	*273/680 = 0.401	0.38
Normal/Near normal scan	5/251 = 0.020	*126/680 = 0.185	0.11
Totals	251	680	

* 150 pts with low probability or normal scans either did not have an angio or the diagnosis of PE was uncertain. On clinical follow-up it was felt that none of these pts had PE. 50 pts with high and intermediate probability scans either did not have an angio or the diagnosis of PE was uncertain. Information on the outcomes of these pts is not included in the paper so it was assumed that they did not have a PE when the above calculations were performed.

Comments

1 50 pts with high and intermediate probability scans did not have angio or the diagnosis of PE was uncertain.

2 Not all pts received gold standard of angio but did get followed up clinically.

PART A — Critical appraisal of a clinical article about prognosis

You see a 70-year old man on outpatient follow-up, three months after his discharge from your hospital with an ischaemic (presumed thrombotic) stroke. He is in sinus rhythm, has mild residual left-sided weakness, but is otherwise well. He had had an upper gastrointestinal bleed while on aspirin a few years earlier, so he is on no medication. His sister-in-law scared him last week by telling him he will probably die by the year's end, and he wants to know what are the chances of this happening to him.

You form the question: 'In a 70-year old man who has had a thrombotic stroke, what is the risk of death within the first year?' You search the *Best Evidence* on disk by typing in 'stroke prognosis' and find 'Mortality in first-ever stroke'. Although it gives you a quick answer – in the form of a structured abstract and clinical commentary – in a few seconds, you soon decide to read the original paper (*Stroke* (1993) **24:** 796–800).

Read the article and decide:
1 Is this evidence about prognosis valid?
2 Is this valid evidence about prognosis important?
3 Can you apply this valid and important evidence about prognosis in caring for your patient?

If you want to read some strategies for answering these sorts of questions, see pp 85–90; 129–132; and 164–165 in *Evidence-based Medicine*.

PART B — Searching the evidence-based journals

We show you how to search the electronic version of two journals: *ACP Journal Club* (*ACPJC*) and *Evidence-based Medicine*. Seven years of the former and two years of the latter are available on disk as *Best Evidence*. This requires a computer with a CD-slot and can be ordered from the BMJ Publishing Group, PO Box 295, London WC1H 9TE; Tel: 0171 387 4499; Fax: 0171 383 6662; e-mail: bmjsubs@dial.pipex.com; or via the website of the Centre for Evidence-based Medicine: http://cebm.jr2.ox.ac.uk/

You could search these evidence-based journals for the answers to some of the questions generated last week.

Now is a good time to start searching on potential topics for your presentations in Sessions 6 and 7.

Long-term Survival After First-Ever Stroke: The Oxfordshire Community Stroke Project

Martin S. Dennis, MD; John P.S. Burn, DM; Peter A.G. Sandercock, DM; John M. Bamford, MD; Derick T. Wade, MD; and Charles P. Warlow, MD

Background and Purpose: There have been relatively few community-based studies of long-term prognosis after acute stroke. This study aimed to provide precise estimates of the absolute and relative risks of dying in an unselected cohort of patients with a first-ever stroke.

Methods: Six hundred seventy-five patients were registered by a community-based stroke register (the Oxfordshire Community Stroke Project) and prospectively followed up for up to 6.5 years. Their relative risk of death was calculated using age- and sex-specific mortality rates for Oxfordshire.

Results: During the first 30 days, 129 (19%) patients died. Patients who survived at least 30 days after a first-ever stroke thereafter had an average annual risk of death of 9.1%, 2.3-fold the risk in people from the general population. Although the absolute (about 15%) and relative (about threefold) risks of death were highest in these 30-day survivors over the first year after the stroke, they were at increased risk of dying over the next few years (range of relative risk for individual years, 1.1–2.9). Predictably, older patients had a worse absolute survival but, relative to the general population, stroke also increased the relative risk of dying in younger patients. During the first 30 days stroke accounts for most deaths; after this time nonstroke cardiovascular disease becomes increasingly important and is the most common cause of death after the first year.

Conclusions: These data highlight the importance of long-term secondary prevention of vascular events in stroke patients, targeted as much at the cardiovascular as at the cerebrovascular circulation. (*Stroke* 1993;24:796–800)

KEY WORDS • epidemiology • Great Britain • prognosis • survival

The risk of death from stroke is highest in the first few weeks after the stroke, although reported 30-day case fatality rates vary widely. Hospital-based studies may report higher early case fatality rates than community-based studies because they include a larger proportion of patients with severe or recurrent strokes, sometimes associated with other nonstroke illnesses. In the Oxfordshire Community Stroke Project (OCSP) the 30-day case fatality rate after a first-ever in a lifetime stroke (first stroke) was 19%.[1] Most of the deaths in the first week resulted from direct damage to the brain, whereas deaths in the subsequent few weeks resulted from complications of immobility (e.g., pneumonia, pulmonary embolism) and less frequently from further vascular events such as recurrent stroke or myocardial infarction.[2] There have been relatively few studies of long-term survival, and even fewer that have

been community based[3–7] and therefore able to report the long-term prognosis of an unselected cohort. In hospital-referred cohorts, the absolute risk of death may be higher and less readily generalizable because referral patterns vary from one hospital to another, and such series are likely to include an unknown and variable excess of patients with severe and recurrent strokes and other illnesses. Alternatively, one might argue that the high early case fatality rate in hospital-referred series may select patients with a good long-term prognosis (i.e., survival effect). Long-term data on the risk of death from all causes, and more specifically deaths from vascular causes, are needed in clinical practice, in the design of clinical trials, and in the planning of health care delivery. In this article we describe the long-term absolute and relative risks of death in an unselected sample of patients with a first stroke in the OCSP.

Methods

Six hundred seventy-five patients with a first stroke were identified prospectively by the OCSP and followed up to establish their long-term prognosis. The study population, clinical definitions, methods employed to ensure complete case ascertainment, methods of assessment, and investigations have been described in detail elsewhere.[8] Surviving patients were followed up by one of two trained research nurses at 1, 6, and 12 months and then annually from the date of stroke onset. At each follow-up visit, the patient was questioned carefully about any symptoms of transient ischemic attack, recur-

From the Department of Clinical Neurosciences (M.S.D., P.A.G.S., C.P.W.), Western General Hospital, Edinburgh; the Department of Rehabilitation Medicine (J.P.S.B.), Southampton General Hospital, Southampton; the Department of Neurology (J.M.B.), St. James's University Hospital, Leeds; and the Rivermead Rehabilitation Centre (D.T.W.), Oxford, U.K.

Supported by the Medical Research Council of Great Britain and the Stroke Association.

Address for correspondence: Dr. Martin S. Dennis, Department of Clinical Neurosciences, Western General Hospital, Edinburgh, U.K., EH4 2XU.

Received December 1, 1992; final revision received January 18, 1993; accepted February 17, 1993.

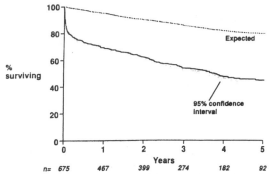

FIGURE 1. *Kaplan-Meier survival curves showing the probability of survival after a first-ever stroke. The shading indicates 95% confidence intervals. The expected survival was calculated from the mortality rates for Oxfordshire, England.[14]*

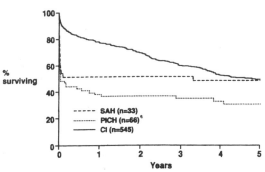

FIGURE 3. *Kaplan-Meier survival curves showing the probability of survival in patients with a first-ever stroke due to cerebral infarction (CI), primary intracerebral hemorrhage (PICH), and subarachnoid hemorrhage (SAH).*

rent stroke, and myocardial infarction; if the nurse suspected that one of these might have occurred, the patient was reassessed by a study neurologist. During 1988 all surviving patients were seen for a more detailed assessment by one of us (J.P.S.B.). When a patient died we reviewed all available hospital, general practitioner, and autopsy records. The cause of death was determined by using all the available clinical evidence rather than just the death certificate, which may be inaccurate.[9,10] For the purposes of this article we classified deaths into five groups: 1) First stroke deaths were due to the direct effects of the brain lesion or due to complications of immobility resulting from the first stroke. These included deaths from bronchopneumonia even several years after the stroke, if stroke-related impairments were thought to be in some way responsible and there was no other, more likely, cause of death. 2) Recurrent stroke deaths were directly due to the brain lesion or complications of immobility following a severe recurrent stroke (i.e., with symptoms that lasted a week or led to early death and were associated with an increase in disability). If deaths from stroke-related impairments occurred after a severe recurrent stroke they were viewed as being due to the recurrent stroke

rather than the first stroke. 3) Cardiovascular deaths were those due to definite or probable cardiac causes, ruptured aortic aneurysm, or peripheral vascular disease. Sudden deaths were regarded as cardiovascular unless an alternative explanation was found at autopsy. 4) Nonvascular deaths were unrelated to any stroke disability and clearly due to a nonvascular cause, e.g., cancer, accidents, or suicide. 5) Unclassified deaths were those in which there was so little information that no cause could be given.

We have described survival using actuarial analysis, in which day 0 was taken as the date of first stroke. Kaplan-Meier survival curves are given with 95% confidence intervals[11] (CIs). The average annual risk of death was calculated by using the method described by Hankey et al.[12] The risk of death for the stroke patients was compared with that for people of similar age and sex from the same general population who were assumed to be stroke free; this was calculated by using the person-years program[13] using age- and sex-specific mortality statistics for Oxfordshire.[14] Approximate 95% CIs of relative risks were calculated using the Poisson distribution.

Results

Six hundred seventy-five patients with a first stroke were identified in the study population during a 4-year

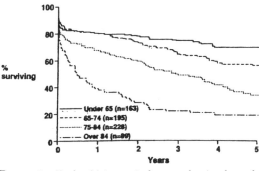

FIGURE 2. *Kaplan-Meier survival curves showing the probability of survival in patients with a first-ever stroke stratified by age. There was a significant trend (χ^2 trend, 75.8; p<0.001) for older patients to have a worse survival.*

TABLE 1. **Relative Risk of Dying After a First-Ever Stroke During Different Time Intervals From Stroke Onset for Patients of All Ages**

Intervals	Number at risk	Observed deaths	Expected deaths	O/E	95% Confidence interval
Year 1	675	208	28.0	7.4	6.5–8.5
Year 2	467	46	24.5	1.9	1.4–2.5
Year 3	399	45	18.0	2.5	1.8–3.4
Year 4	274	31	14.3	2.2	1.5–3.1
Year 5	182	8	7.1	1.1	0.5–2.2
Year 6	92	9	3.2	2.9	1.3–5.4
30 days–6 years	546	218	93.1	2.3	2.0–2.7
All intervals	675	347	95.0	3.7	3.3–4.1

O/E, observed deaths/expected deaths.

TABLE 2. Relative Risk of Dying After a First-Ever Stroke in Patients of Different Ages for All Time Intervals

Age	Number at risk	Observed deaths	Expected deaths	O/E	95% Confidence interval
<45 years	26	3	0.1	37.5	6.2–87.7
45–54 years	25	8	0.3	25.8	11.1–50.8
55–64 years	112	32	3.0	10.6	7.3–14.9
65–74 years	195	75	15.6	4.8	3.8–6.0
75–84 years	228	145	44.3	3.3	2.8–3.9
>84 years	89	84	31.8	2.7	2.1–3.3
All ages	675	347	95.0	3.7	3.3–4.1

O/E, observed deaths/expected deaths.

period. Their mean age was 72 years; 318 (47%) were male. The pathological type of the first stroke was cerebral infarction in 545 (81%), primary intracerebral hemorrhage in 66 (10%), subarachnoid hemorrhage in 33 (5%), and unknown pathological type in 31 (5%). Surviving patients were followed up for a minimum of 2 years and up to 6.5 years. By the end of the follow-up period, 347 (51%) patients had died. An autopsy was conducted in 56 (43%) of the 129 patients dying in the first 30 days, but in only 44 (20%) of the 218 dying thereafter. No patient was lost to follow-up.

Absolute Risks for All Patients

A Kaplan-Meier survival curve for all 675 patients is shown in Figure 1. The risks of death over the first 30 days and over the first year were about 19% (95% CI, 16–22%) and 31% (95% CI, 27–34%), respectively. For those surviving at least 30 days or for at least 1 year, the average annual risks of death up to 5 years were 9.1% (95% CI, 8.1–10.4%) and 6.6% (95% CI, 4.6–8.8%), respectively. In 30-day survivors the risk of dying was higher in the remainder of the first year (about 15%) than in subsequent years.

Absolute Risks for Subgroups

Stratification by age showed that older patients had a worse prognosis (χ^2 trend, 75.8; $p<0.001$), both during the early period after the stroke and throughout the follow-up period (Figure 2). There was a nonsignificant trend for women to have a worse prognosis than men, but this disappeared after correcting for differences in age (age-adjusted relative odds, M:F=0.93; 95% CI, 0.74–1.15%). The survival curves comparing prognosis in the different pathological types of stroke are shown in Figure 3. As we have demonstrated previously,[1] the

survival curves diverge over the first 30 days but, because few ($n=50$) patients with intracranial hemorrhage survived beyond 30 days, comparisons of late survival are unreliable, although the long-term risk of death after primary intracerebral hemorrhage did see similar to the risk after cerebral infarction. The risk of dying in the first year after a first stroke due to cerebral infarction was 22.1% (95% CI, 18.9–26.9%). In cerebral infarction patients who were alive at the end of the first year, the average annual risk of death over the next 4 years was 8.5% (95% CI, 6.1–10.5%). The long-term prognosis for 30-day survivors of subarachnoid hemorrhage was good, with only two of 18 survivors dying subsequently, which may reflect their relatively young age and the protective effect of aneurysm surgery.

Relative Risk Compared With General Population

The risk of dying after a first stroke compared with the risk of death in people of similar age and sex in the general population is shown in Tables 1 and 2. The relative risk is given for each yearly interval from the onset of stroke (Table 1) and for different age bands (Table 2). In the first year stroke patients had a 7.4-fold risk (95% CI, 6.5–8.5%) of death varying between 1.1 and 2.9 in subsequent years. Patients who survived at least 30 days had approximately a threefold greater risk of dying in the next year than people in the general population. The relative risk was far greater in younger patients. In the first year the relative risk of dying in a 45–54-year-old was 71.8 (95% CI, 27.5–163.3%) compared with a relative risk for all ages in the first year of 7.4 (95% CI, 6.5–8.5%). In the second and third years, the relative risk of dying in younger patients remained higher, though this was based on very few deaths (two in the 45–54-year-old age group), so that we cannot be certain whether younger survivors of stroke have continuing increased risk of dying compared with stroke-free individuals. The relative risk for all stroke patients of all ages was 3.7 over the first 6 years, and for those surviving 30 days the subsequent relative risk was 2.3 (95% CI, 2.0–2.7%). For all ages combined, the relative risk of death over the first year after cerebral infarction (all ages) was 4.8 (95% CI, 4.2–5.7%) and 2.1 (95% CI, 1.8–2.5%) over the next 5 years.

Causes of Death

Table 3 and Figure 4 show the causes of death during different time intervals from the onset of the first stroke. For those patients who survived at least 30 days, 36% of subsequent deaths were due to the first or recurrent

TABLE 3. Causes of Death Within Different Time Intervals After a First-Ever Stroke

	Number of deaths within each time interval								
Causes of death	0–30 days *n*	30 Days–6 months *n*	6 Months–1 year *n*	1–2 Years *n*	2–3 Years *n*	3–4 Years *n*	4–5 Years *n*	5–6 Years *n*	All intervals
First stroke	116 (90)	22 (44)	8 (28)	5 (11)	3 (7)	1 (3)	0 (0)	2 (22)	157
Recurrent stroke	1 (1)	9 (18)	6 (21)	7 (15)	5 (11)	8 (26)	0 (0)	2 (22)	38
Nonstroke/ cardiovascular	9 (7)	11 (22)	9 (31)	24 (56)	10 (22)	14 (45)	3 (38)	4 (44)	84
Nonvascular	3 (2)	8 (16)	5 (17)	9 (20)	26 (58)	8 (26)	4 (50)	1 (11)	64
Unknown	0 (0)	0 (0)	1 (3)	1 (2)	1 (2)	0 (0)	1 (12)	0 (0)	4
All causes	129	50	29	46	45	31	8	9	347

Numbers in parentheses are percent of deaths.

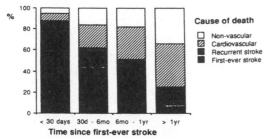

FIGURE 4. *Histogram showing the proportion of patients dying from different causes during different time intervals from the onset of their first-ever stroke.*

stroke, whereas 34% were due to other vascular causes. Of the patients who survived at least 30 days after their first stroke due to cerebral infarction but who then died during the follow-up period, 33 (17%) died of their first stroke, 32 (16%) died as a result of recurrent stroke, 70 (35%) died of a nonstroke cardiovascular cause, and 60 (30%) died of nonvascular causes. In four (2%) the cause of death was unknown. Among the patients with primary intracerebral hemorrhage, subarachnoid hemo rhage, and unknown pathology, there were only 19 deaths after 30 days, so that no conclusions could be drawn from these data.

Conclusions

This study is important because it is community-based and therefore provides an unselected series of first-stroke patients for study; there was a prospective neurological assessment; a large proportion of stroke patients underwent a CT scan or autopsy to determine th: pathological type of stroke; follow-up was prospective and prolonged; and it provides estimates of relative as well as absolute risks. Table 4 shows the only other studies that were community based and have published long-term (at least 5-year) survival data.

The risk of dying over the first 5 years after stroke is similar in the different studies and is probably not statistically significantly different except for that from Moscow,[3] where 72% (95% CI, 70–74%) of the study subjects died compared with risks of 45% (95% CI, 37.7–51.5%)[4] to 61% (95% CI, 51.4–70.6%)[6] in the other studies. (Scmidt et al[3] gave the actual rather than the actuarial risk, although this was comparable because all patients appear to have been followed up for at least 5 years or until death.) This poorer survival may have been, in part, because the Moscow study[3] included recurrent strokes in their inception cohort. The study with the next worse prognosis[6] may also have included recurrent strokes in their inception cohort. Perhaps of more interest is the relative risk of dying in stroke patients compared with people in the general population in the different studies. Our study suggests that patients have a persistent and statistically significant excess risk of death for several years after their first stroke. Sacco et al,[4] using data from the Framingham study, also demonstrated that the excess risk of dying persists for several years, although those without coexistent hypertension or heart disease had no excess risk if they survived the first year. This suggested to the authors that any excess risk of death was related to such coexistent problems rather than to the stroke itself. Data from Rochester, Minnesota[15] suggested that patients who had survived at least a year after a stroke had little or no excess risk of death in subsequent years; there may have been several methodological reasons for this difference, but the most likely is simply the small number of patients and the very small number of deaths, which gave imprecise estimates of relative risk. Failure to show a significant excess of deaths after year 1 may have been a false-negative (type 2) error. Indeed, these previous studies have not provided any measure of the precision of their results. Even in our study the estimates of excess risk were fairly imprecise (see 95% CIs in Tables 1 and 2).

TABLE 4. Comparison of Risk of Death After Stroke in Community-Based Studies

Study	Diagnosis	Actuarial risk of death (%)		
		30 Days	By 1 year	By 5 years
OCSP	Cerebral infarction	10	23	52
	PICH	52	62	70
	SAH	45	48	52
	All first-ever strokes	19	31	45
Framingham[4]	Cerebral infarction	15	NA	NA
	PICH	82	NA	NA
	SAH	46	NA	NA
	All first-ever strokes	22	NA	Men 48
				Women 40
Rochester[15]	Cerebral infarction	16	NA	52
	PICH	58	NA	NA
	SAH	37	NA	NA
	All first-ever strokes	23	39	54
Moscow[3]	All strokes	37	52	72
Ikawa[6]	All strokes	NA	32	61

OCSP, Oxfordshire Community Stroke Project; PICH, primary intracerebral hemorrhage; SAH, subarachnoid hemorrhage; NA, not available.

800   **Stroke** *Vol 24, No 6 June 1993*

Our data confirm that the risk of death early after a first stroke is high, which supports the worldwide efforts to identify medical treatments to improve early prognosis. Although deaths due to stroke are proportionally the most important early on, in subsequent years deaths due to recurrent stroke and in particular those due to cardiovascular problems become numerically more important. The finding that stroke patients have a significant excess risk of death even after the first year demonstrates a clear need for prolonged secondary prevention aimed equally at the heart and cerebral circulations.

Acknowledgments

We wish to thank all those who have helped with this project, including Sue Price, Liz Mogridge, and Claire Clifford, our study nurses; Lesley Jones, the project computer programmer; and Helen Storrie, Venessa Langsbury, Angie Dwyer, and Andrea Watts, who provided secretarial support. We especially thank our collaborating general practitioners, without whom this project would be impossible. The collaborating practices were (name of liaison partner from each practice only): Dr. A. MacPherson, Oxford; Dr. A. Marcus, Thames; Dr. D. Leggate, Oxford; Dr. M. Agass, Berinsfield; Dr. D. Otterburn, Abingdon; Dr. S. Street, Kidlington; Dr. V. Drury, Wantage; Dr. R. Pinches, Abingdon; Dr. N. Crossley, Abingdon; and Dr. H. O'Donnell, Deddington.

References

1. Bamford J, Sandercock P, Dennis M, Burn J, Warlow C: A prospective study of acute cerebrovascular disease in the community: The Oxfordshire Community Stroke Project—1981–1986: 2. Incidence, case fatality rates and overall outcome at one year of cerebral infarction, primary intracerebral and subarachnoid haemorrhage. *J Neurol Neurosurg Psychiatry* 1990;53:16–22
2. Bamford J, Dennis M, Sandercock P, Burn J, Warlow C: The frequency, causes and timing of death within 30 days of a first stroke: The Oxfordshire Community Stroke Project. *J Neurol Neurosurg Psychiatry* 1990;53:824–829
3. Scmidt EV, Smirnov VE, Ryabova VS: Results of the seven-year prospective study of stroke patients. *Stroke* 1988;19:942–949
4. Sacco RL, Wolf PA, Kannel WB, McNamara PM: Survival and recurrence following stroke: The Framingham study. *Stroke* 1982; 13:290–296
5. Matsumoto N, Whisnant JP, Kurland LT, Okazaki H: Natural history of stroke in Rochester, Minnesota, 1955 through 1969: An extension of a previous study, 1945 through 1954. *Stroke* 1973;4: 20–29
6. Kojima S, Omura T, Wakamatsu W, Kishi M, Yamazaki T, Iida M, Komachi Y: Prognosis and disability of stroke patients after 5 Years in Akita, Japan. *Stroke* 1990;21:72–77
7. Garraway WM, Whisnant JP, Drury I: The changing pattern of survival following stroke. *Stroke* 1983;14:699–703
8. Bamford J, Sandercock P, Dennis M, Warlow C, Jones L, MacPherson K, Vessey M, Fowler G, Molyneux A, Hughes T, Burn J, Wade D: A prospective study of acute cerebrovascular disease in the community: The Oxfordshire Community Stroke Project—1981–1986: 1. Methodology, demography and incidence cases of first-ever stroke. *J Neurol Neurosurg Psychiatry* 1988;51: 1373–1380
9. Cameron HM, McGoogan E: A prospective study of 1152 hospital autopsies: 1. Inaccuracies in death certification. *J Pathol* 1981;133: 273–283
10. Cameron HM, McGoogan E: A prospective study of 1152 hospital autopsies: 2. Analysis of inaccuracies in clinical diagnosis and their significance. *J Pathol* 1981;133:285–300
11. Machin D, Gardner MJ: Calculating confidence intervals for survival time analyses, in Gardner MJ, Altman DG (eds): *Statistics With Confidence.* Belfast, *Br Med J,* 1989, pp 64–70
12. Hankey GJ, Slattery JM, Warlow CP: The prognosis of hospital referred transient ischaemic attacks. *J Neurol Neurosurg Psychiatry* 1991;54:793–802
13. Coleman M, Douglas A, Herman C, Peto J: Cohort study analysis with a fortran computer program. *Int J Epidemiol* 1986;15:134–137
14. Office of Population, Census and Surveys: *Mortality Statistics 1985.* London, Her Majesty's Stationery Office, 1987
15. Dyken ML: Natural history of ischaemic stroke in cerebrovascular disease, in Harrison MJG, Dyken ML (eds): *Butterworth International Medical Reviews: Neurology,* ed 3. London, Butterworth, 1983, pp 139–170

Citation:

Are the results of this prognosis study valid?

Was a defined, representative sample of patients
assembled at a common (usually early) point in
the course of their disease?

Was patient follow up sufficiently long and
complete?

Were objective outcome criteria applied in a
'blind' fashion?

If subgroups with different prognoses are
identified, was there adjustment for important
prognostic factors?

Was there validation in an independent group
('test-set') of patients?

Are the valid results of this prognosis study important?

How likely are the outcomes over time?

How precise are the prognostic estimates?

If you want to calculate a confidence interval around the measure of prognosis

(*see* Appendix 1 in *Evidence-based Medicine*.)

Clinical Measure	Standard Error (SE)	Typical calculation of CI
Proportion (as in the rate of some prognostic event, etc.) where: the number of patients = n the proportion of these patients who experience the event = p	$\sqrt{\{p \times (1-p) / n\}}$ where p is proportion and n is number of patients	If $p = 24/60 = 0.4$ (or 40%) and $n=60$ $SE = \sqrt{\{0.4 \times (1-0.4) / 60\}}$ $= 0.063$ (or 6.3%) 95% CI is 40% +/– 1.96 x 6.3% or 27.6% to 52.4%
n from your evidence: _____ p from your evidence: _____	$\sqrt{\{p \times (1-p) / n\}}$ where p is proportion and n is number of patients	Your calculation: SE: _____ 95% CI: _____

Can you apply this valid, important evidence about prognosis in caring for your patient?

Is your patient so different from those in the study that its results can't help you?

Will this evidence make a clinically important impact on your conclusions about what to offer or tell your patient?

Additional notes

Citation: Dennis MS, Burn JP, Sandercock PA, *et al*. (1993) Long-term survival after first-ever stroke: The Oxfordshire Community Stroke Project. *Stroke.* 24: 796-800.

Are the results of this prognosis study valid?

Was a defined, representative sample of patients assembled at a common (usually early) point in the course of their disease?	**Yes. From a common starting point but we don't know how GPs decided which stroke patients to send to hospital.**
Was patient follow up sufficiently long and complete?	**Yes. For a minimum of 2 years and up to 6.5 years.**
Were objective outcome criteria applied in a 'blind' fashion?	**Objective outcome criteria were applied but observations were not blinded.**
If subgroups with different prognoses are identified, was there adjustment for important prognostic factors?	**Some stratification by age and type of stroke, but not for clinically relevant subgroups (these are reported in a later paper: *Stroke* (1994) 25: 333–337).**
Was there validation in an independent group ('test-set') of patients?	**No.**

Are the valid results of this prognosis study important?

How likely are the outcomes over time?	**The estimate for our patient dying in the first year after a cerebral infarction was 22%, but because he's already survived the first month's high risk, his chance of dying in the remainder of the first year are less than half that.**
How precise are the prognostic estimates?	**The 95% confidence interval on that 22% runs from 19% to 27%, so it's pretty precise.**

If you want to calculate a confidence interval around the measure of prognosis

(*see* Appendix 1 in *Evidence-based Medicine*.)

Clinical Measure	Standard Error (SE)	Typical calculation of CI
Proportion (as in the rate of some prognostic event, etc.) where:	$\sqrt{\{p \times (1-p) / n\}}$ where p is proportion and n is number of patients	If p = 24/60 = 0.4 (or 40%) and n=60
the number of patients = n		SE = $\sqrt{\{0.4 \times (1-0.4) / 60\}}$ = 0.063 (or 6.3%)
the proportion of these patients who experience the event = p		95% CI is 40% +/– 1.96 x 6.3% or 27.6% to 52.4%
n from your evidence: **675** p from your evidence: **0.22**	$\sqrt{\{p \times (1-p) / n\}}$ where p is proportion and n is number of patients	Your calculation: SE: **0.016** 95% CI: **+/– 3%**

Can you apply this valid, important evidence about prognosis in caring for your patient?

Is your patient so different from those in the study that its results can't help you?	**Yes.**
Will this evidence make a clinically important impact on your conclusions about what to offer or tell your patient?	**In this patient, yes.**

Additional notes

For clinical subgroups, see *Stroke* (1994) 25: 333–337.

Clinical Bottom Line

A patient with an ischaemic stroke, who is not on any antiplatelet agents or anticoagulants and is otherwise well, has a 22% risk of dying within the first year.

Citation

Denis MS, Burn JP, Sandercock PA, *et al.* (1993) Long-term survival after first-ever stroke: The Oxfordshire Community Stroke Project. *Stroke.* **24:** 796–800.

Clinical Question

In a patient with thrombotic stroke, what is the risk of death within the first year?

Search Terms

'stroke prognosis' in *Best Evidence.*

The Study

Cohort of 675 patients registered in a community-based stroke registry followed up prospectively for up to 6.5 years.

The Evidence

Group	Event	Timing	Rate	95% C.I.
Ischaemic strokes	Death	One year	22%	19% to 27%
All strokes	Death	One month	19%	16% to 22%
All strokes	Death	One year	31%	27% to 34%
All strokes who survived first year	Death	Annual death rate for years 2–5	6.6%	4.6% to 8.8%

Comments

1 Unsure how physicians selected patients for registration.

2 Not all potentially important prognostic factors adjusted for, e.g. antiplatelet therapy, use of anticoagulants, a fib and size of the left atrium.

3 Outcome observers were not blinded.

4 Some outcome events were not picked up until the next follow up visit, which could have been up to a year after the event – investigators had to rely on patient information and medical records in that case.

5 For subgroups, see later paper: *Stroke* (1994) **25:** 333–7.

STROKE – PROGNOSIS AT ONE YEAR

Appraised by Sharon Straus, October 1996.
Expiry date: 1998.

SOURCES OF EVIDENCE FOR EVIDENCE-BASED MEDICINE

Title	Medium	Content type	Advantages	Disadvantages
Best Evidence **on Disk (American College of Physicians & BMJ Publications Group)**	CD-ROM or diskette (cumulated contents of two paper journals: *ACP Journal Club* and *Evidence-based Medicine*.) Updated every year.	Structured abstracts of articles from selected journals in internal medicine, general practice, obstetrics and gynaecology, paediatrics, psychiatry, and surgery. Articles must meet strict quality criteria; each abstract (evidence) accompanied by a commentary (clinical expertise).	High quality evidence with commentary; easy to search; high specificity (not much time wasted with irrelevant material)	Incomplete coverage of literature: low sensitivity.

WHEN TO USE IT: *As your first port of call for the specialities it covers.*

Title	Medium	Content type	Advantages	Disadvantages
Cochrane Library	CD-ROM or diskette or Internet	Superb evidence about therapy and prevention; >100 world-wide systematic reviews; >1,000 abstracts of overviews of effectiveness.	Highest quality evidence we'll ever have on the effectiveness of health care.	Not yet many Cochrane reviews; necessarily omits the newest treatments.

WHEN TO USE IT: *As your best port of call for therapy.*

Title	Medium	Content type	Advantages	Disadvantages
MEDLINE (US National Library of Medicine)	Networked CD-ROM systems; on-line vendors. (SilverPlatter [WinSPIRS] Ovid, etc.)	Bibliographic records, with abstract and MeSH terms. Full-text services starting to appear.	Exhaustiveness; flexibility of searching; journal coverage; currency (on-line versions); widespread availability and support (lots of people can help you!)	Have to do your own quality filtering; putting together good searches is difficult; gaps in coverage (medical, geographical and linguistic).

WHEN TO USE IT: *When you need to be sure you've got everything and have time to search properly.*

Title	Medium	Content type	Advantages	Disadvantages
World-Wide Web (WWW)	Internet (via browser programs such as Netscape, MS Internet Explorer, Mosaic, Yahoo, Lynx, etc.)	Everything: from LRs to NNTs; electronic journals (e.g. Bandolier) and journal clubs; software tools; CATs; teaching materials; searching tips; events and conferences; etc.	Some sites are excellent, with high-quality pre-filtered evidence; some good, free software; boundless possibilities; can be updated instantly.	Variable levels of quality control; poor sensitivity and specificity; access from NHS networks can be problematic; can be slow to download.

WHEN TO USE IT: *Find good sites and check them regularly for updates.*

Title	Medium	Content type	Advantages	Disadvantages
Recommended sites:	CEBM	http://cebm.jr2.ox.ac.uk/	CATs, NNTs, LRs, etc., teaching materials, announcements, links to other sites.	
	SCHARR / AurACLE	http://panizzi.shef.ac.uk/auracle/aurac.html	Evidence-based information seeking, links to other sites.	
	Bandolier	http://www.jr2.ox.ac.uk/Bandolier/	An electronic version (including back issues) of the EBM journal *Bandolier*.	
WWW search services	General comment on Web searching	Allows you to type in keywords and search an index of WWW pages.	Tens of millions of pages are indexed and can be accessed directly. Searching is crude and hits displayed in an order which is not always appropriate.	
Typical specific services:	Yahoo!	http://www.yahoo.com	More selective than most search sites, though this may not coincide with your needs!	
	AltaVista	http://www.altavista.com	Seems to be the most exhaustive, with best searching engine.	

WHEN TO USE IT: *To find very specific information from the Web or starting points for browsing.*

EBM SESSION

4

SECTION 1

Systematic
reviews &
searching
the primary
literature

PART A — Critical appraisal of a systematic review about thrombolytic therapy.

It is a typically busy night 'on take' and you are working up a fascinating (but impatient) individual with dark (bronzed?) skin, hepatomegaly and diabetes (with two 'pneumonias', a 'stroke' and three 'confused' waiting in the wings) when the A & E room bleeps you to report that another patient (a 55-year old taxi driver) has been admitted with a possible myocardial infarction (he drove himself to hospital during his first-ever episode of crushing chest pain, and arrived within 25 minutes of its inception). He is haemodynamically stable, his ECG is judged to show clear-cut ST-elevation in 3 anterior leads, and he has no contraindications to thrombolysis. They are pushing you to drop everything and rush over and 'lyse him, but you'd rather continue the work-up for haemochromatosis.

Grudgingly, you comply with their request, confirm that the cabby is a candidate for thrombolysis, and treat him with streptokinase and aspirin. By the time you get back to your bronzed patient, he has left.

You wonder just how important it was for you to drop everything to initiate thrombolysis during the first hour of symptoms, and form the question: 'In a patient who deserves thrombolytic therapy for presumed myocardial infarction, does the initiation of treatment within the first hour (rather than waiting an hour) really lead to clinically important lower mortality?' A search of *Best Evidence* using 'thrombolysis' and 'myocardial infarction' finds an article that looks potentially very useful (*Lancet* (1996) **348:** 771–5).

Read the systematic review and decide:
1   Is this evidence from this systematic review valid?
2   Is this valid evidence from this systematic review important?
3   Can you apply this valid and important evidence from this systematic review in caring for your patient?

If you want to read some strategies for answering these sorts of questions, see pp 97–99; 140–141 and 166–172 in *Evidence-based Medicine*.

PART B — Searching for evidence in the primary literature

Colleagues from the library will come and whet your appetite for learning how to search for evidence in the clinical literature or hone the searching skills you already have developed. So bring along the clinical questions you generated in Session 2 (or any that you have generated in the meantime). Efficient EBM searching strategies that trade-off the sensitivity and specificity of your searches are on the next page.

If you haven't already done your search for your presentation in Sessions 6 and 7, now would be a good time to do it!

BEST SINGLE TERMS AND COMBINATIONS FOR HIGH SENSITIVITY MEDLINE SEARCHES ON THE BEST STUDIES OF TREATMENT, DIAGNOSIS, PROGNOSIS, OR CAUSE

Search strategy	Sensitivity[1]	Specificity	Precision
For studies of treatment:			
Clinical trial (pt)	0.93	0.92	0.49
Randomised controlled trial (pt) or Drug therapy (sh) or Therapeutic use (sh) or Random: (tw)	0.99	0.74	0.22
For studies of prognosis:			
Exp cohort studies	0.60	0.80	0.11
Incidence or Exp mortality or Follow up studies or Mortality: (sh) or Prognosis: (tw) or Predict: (tw) or Course: (tw)	0.92	0.73	0.11
For studies of aetiology or cause:			
Risk (tw)	0.67	0.79	0.15
Exp cohort studies or Exp risk or Odds and ratio: (tw) or Relative and risk: (tw) or Case and control: (tw)	0.82	0.70	0.14
For studies of diagnosis:			
Diagnosis (pe)	0.80	0.77	0.09
Exp Sensitivity and specificity or Diagnosis: (pe) or Diagnostic use or Sensitivity: (tw) or Specificity: (tw)	0.92	0.73	0.09

[1]**Sensitivity**, as defined in the study on which the table is based, is the proportion of studies in MEDLINE meeting criteria for scientific soundness and clinical relevance that are detected. **Specificity** is the proportion of less sound/relevant studies that are excluded by the search strategy. **Precision** is the proportion of all citations retrieved that are both sound and relevant. (Source: *Evidence-based Medicine*; also see the Web pages.)

Articles

Early thrombolytic treatment in acute myocardial infarction: reappraisal of the golden hour

Eric Boersma, Arthur C P Maas, Jaap W Deckers, Maarten L Simoons

Summary

Background There is conclusive evidence from clinical trials that reduction of mortality by fibrinolytic therapy in acute myocardial infarction is related to the time elapsing between onset of symptoms and commencement of treatment. However, the exact pattern of this relation continues to be debated. This paper discusses whether or not appreciable additional gain can be achieved with very early treatment.

Methods The relation between treatment delay and short-term mortality (up to 35 days) was evaluated using tabulated data from all randomised trials of at least 100 patients (n=22; 50 246 patients) that compared fibrinolytic therapy with placebo or control, reported between 1983 and 1993.

Findings Benefit of fibrinolytic therapy was 65 (SD 14), 37 (9), 26 (6) and 29 (5) lives saved per 1000 treated patients in the 0–1, 1–2, 2–3, and 3–6 h intervals, respectively. Proportional mortality reduction was significantly higher in patients treated within 2 h compared to those treated later (44% [95% CI 32, 53] vs 20% [15, 25]; p=0·001). The relation between treatment delay and mortality reduction per 1000 treated patients was expressed significantly better by a non-linear ($19\cdot4 - 0\cdot6x + 29\cdot3x^{-1}$) than a linear ($34\cdot7 - 1\cdot6x$) regression equation (p=0·03).

Interpretation The beneficial effect of fibrinolytic therapy is substantially higher in patients presenting within 2 h after symptom onset compared to those presenting later.

Lancet 1996; **348**: 771–75

Erasmus University, Rotterdam, Netherlands (E Boersma MSc, A C P Maas MD, Prof J W Deckers MD, Prof M L Simoons PhD)

Correspondence to: Prof M L Simoons, Thoraxcenter Bd 434, Erasmus University and University Hospital Rotterdam-Dijkzigt, Dr Molewaterplein 40, 3015 GD Rotterdam, Netherlands

Introduction

The reduction in mortality that can be achieved with reperfusion therapy in patients with evolving myocardial infarction depends on the time elapsing between onset of symptoms and initiation of treatment or, more specifically, on the duration of coronary occlusion before reperfusion.[1] Although earlier reperfusion yields a better clinical outcome the relation between treatment delay and mortality reduction is controversial. A key question is whether or not a substantial additional reduction of the mortality risk can be achieved with very early treatment, ie, within 2–3 h after onset of symptoms. The concept of a 'first golden hour'[2] is supported both by experimental studies and randomised trials comparing pre-hospital with in-hospital therapy.[2,3] By contrast, the Fibrinolytic Therapy Trialists' (FTT) Collaborative Group, in a pooled dataset of randomised trials of more than 1000 patients,[4] reported only a gradual decrease of benefit with longer delay. We present an alternative analysis of data from previous trials.

Experimental studies

The duration of coronary occlusion and the extent of collateral circulation are the main determinants of infarct size in pigs, dogs, cats, and other animals.[5-7] In animals with a coronary collateral circulation similar to that of humans an occlusion persisting for 15–30 min generally does not lead to significant myocardial damage.[6,7] Thus, necrosis can be prevented provided reperfusion is achieved within this period.[8] A small area of necrosis usually occurs with reperfusion after 45 min occlusion, while the mid-endocardial and subendocardial zones are still viable.[6] Longer durations of coronary occlusion result in progressive growth of the infarction and reduction of the amount of salvageable myocardium. At 90 min the extent of cell death involves 40–50% of the area at risk; less than half of the jeopardised myocardium remains viable at that time.[3,8] 6 h after the onset of continuous ischaemia the area at risk is fully infarcted such that myocardial salvage will be minimal.

In humans, the thrombotic event frequently consists of multiple cycles of temporary occlusion and reperfusion. The degree of chest pain (if present) varies among patients so that it is often difficult to determine the exact duration of the coronary occlusion. Nevertheless, data indicate that evolution of (enzymatically detectable) infarct size over time in humans shows a pattern similar to that in animals.[9]

Pre-hospital versus in-hospital thrombolysis

Various clinical trials have shown that early restoration of coronary patency improves survival.[10-13] Later recanalisation may also be beneficial, particularly in patients with sufficient collateral flow and in those with stuttering infarction. Randomised trials comparing pre-

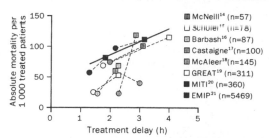

Figure 1: **Mortality at 35 days in randomised studies comparing prehospital (circles) with inhospital (squares) thrombolytic therapy**

All trials (except that of Castaigne) showed trend favouring prehospital thrombolysis. Regression line (bold, weighted by number of patients included in mortality result) was mainly determined by EMIP study.

hospital with in-hospital therapy[14-21] have shown a substantial beneficial effect of very early thrombolytic therapy. Although these studies were too small to show statistical significance, such significance was reached in pooled analyses of the data.[2,22] The largest EMIP trial, with 5469 randomised patients, reported 15 (SD 8) additional patients alive at 30 days per 1000 patients as a result of 1 h earlier treatment.[21] Figure 1 shows the weighted regression line of all eight randomised studies.[14-21] In these studies, the average delay from symptom onset to initiation of therapy was 2·1 h in the prehospital patients and 3·1 h in the inhospital patients. 1 h earlier treatment within 3 h from symptom onset is associated with a benefit of 21 (6) lives per 1000 treated (p=0·002).

FTT analysis

The Fibrinolytic Therapy Trialists' Collaborative Group presented a systematic analysis of the pooled data from all unconfounded trials of fibrinolytic therapy *versus* control or placebo that randomised at least 1000 patients with suspected myocardial infarction.[4] Nine trials were included with 58 600 patients, among whom 6177 deaths (10·5%) were reported within 35 days. The effect of treatment on mortality and morbidity was studied in various patient categories. One of the FTT subanalyses described the benefits of fibrinolytic therapy in five subgroups according to the delay from symptom onset to randomisation (0–1, ≥1–3, ≥3–6, ≥6–12 and ≥12–24 h). Mortality reduction was highest among patients presenting in hospital within 1 h: the absolute benefit was 35 (11) additional patients alive per 1000 treated. In patients presenting ≥1–3 and ≥3–6 h the benefits were 25 (5) and 19 (5) additional alive patients per 1000 treated, respectively.

In patients with ST elevation or bundle branch block (n=45 000, 77% of the population) the absolute effects of fibrinolytic therapy were slightly larger. Benefits per 1000 treated patients were 39 (12), 30 (5), 27 (6), 21 (7), and 7 (7) in the respective subgroups. The relation between these benefits and the average delay from symptom onset (0·98, 2·50, 4·79, 9·11, and 17·48 h, respectively) was described as a straight regression line. Every additional hour of treatment delay from onset of symptoms was associated with a reduction in benefit by approximately 1·6 (0·6) lives per 1000 patients.

The FTT investigators concluded from these data a gradually increasing benefit with earlier treatment, without significant additional treatment effect at 0–1 h. According

to this analysis little would be gained by extra efforts to achieve very early, prehospital, therapy.

Alternative presentation of trial data

Since the FTT analysis is at variance with the experimental data, and with the larger benefit found in direct, randomised comparison of prehospital with inhospital therapy, an alternative presentation of the trial data seems appropriate. Furthermore, estimations of benefit for early treatment in the FTT analysis may have been influenced by the chosen framework for analysis.

The inclusion-threshold of 1000 patients for each of the nine studies included in the FTT analysis is rather arbitrary. There is no good reason to exclude smaller trials. Although the number of patients in the smaller studies may not be sufficient to prove the effect of thrombolytic therapy, these studies may nevertheless assist a more powerful estimation of treatment effects in subgroups of patients in a pooled dataset; more so, because several smaller studies excluded from the FTT analysis included a significant proportion of patients who were treated very early.

The statistical analysis was based on subdivision of patients according to delay from symptom onset with only two benefit estimations in the first 3 h (at average delay times of 0·98 and 2·50 h, respectively). In this way, part of a potential large effect in the first 2 h may be obscured by a relatively small effect in the third hour. A more differentiated subdivision seems more appropriate to study the effect of very early therapy.[2] Furthermore, non-linear models might be developed and tested in addition to the linear FTT model.

Methods

For the reasons given, we studied the delay/benefit relation in a modified dataset, covering all randomised trials of fibrinolytic therapy *versus* placebo or control which included at least 100 patients. These trials were reported between 1983 and 1993 and indexed in the MEDLINE information system.[24] There are 22 such trials[12,13,25-44] The indication for fibrinolytic therapy in two of the trials may not have been appropriate: the USIM trial included a high proportion (32%) of patients with unstable angina, and the ISIS-3 uncertain indication group consisted of patients without or with only minor ST elevation;[43,44] these patient subgroups are unlikely to benefit from fibrinolysis.[45-47] The USIM and ISIS-3 trials included 4250 patients who were treated within 3 h of symptom onset and may therefore seriously bias benefit estimations for early treatment of those with confirmed infarction. Accordingly, we analysed data from previous trials both with and without inclusion of USIM and the ISIS-3 uncertain indication group.

Tabulated data were collected on time from symptom onset and short-term mortality (up to 35 days). Mortality observations of the separate trials were positioned at the average treatment delay, if reported, and otherwise at the mid-point of the described time-window. The data of 11 trials were sufficiently detailed to be split into different time intervals.[12,13,27,29,31-33,41-44] Patients were subsequently allocated to six subgroups according to treatment delay (0–1, ≥1–2, ≥2–3, ≥3–6, ≥6–12, and ≥12–24 h from symptom onset to randomisation). Absolute and relative mortality effects of fibrinolytic therapy were evaluated in each of these categories. USIM and ISIS-3 uncertain indication patients were excluded from this analysis.

Benefit was defined as the absolute mortality reduction, calculated as the difference in the percentage dying in the fibrinolytic group and the controls (we also calculated the SD and 95% CI of this difference). Linear $(\alpha+\beta x)$ and non-linear $(\alpha+\beta x+\gamma x^2$ and $\alpha+\beta x+\gamma x^{-1})$ regression analyses were performed to determine the relation between benefit and treatment delay.

Session 4 – Systematic reviews & searching the primary literature

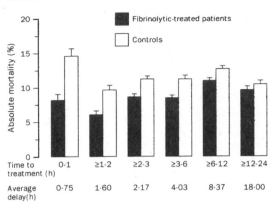

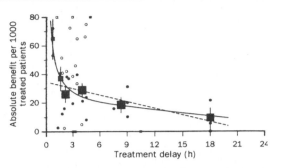

Figure 4: **Absolute 35-day mortality reduction versus treatment delay**

Small closed dots: information from trials included in FTT analysis; open dots: information from additional trials; small squares: data beyond scale of x/y cross. The linear (34·7–1·6x) and non-linear (19·4–0·6x+29·3x⁻¹) regression lines are fitted within these data, weighted by inverse of the variance of the absolute benefit in each datapoint.[4] Black squares: average effects in six time-to-treatment groups (areas of squares inversely proportional to variance of absolute benefit described).

Figure 2: **Mortality at 35 days among fibrinolytic-treated and control patients, according to treatment delay**

Regression functions were fitted in the tabulated data from the separate trials. Data were weighted by the inverse of the variance of the absolute benefit described.[4] Goodness of fit was expressed as the ratio of regression sum of squares and total sum of squares (R^2-value). Regression analyses were performed both with and without USIM and ISIS-3 uncertain indication data.

Results

The 22 trials included a total of 50 246 patients, of whom 5762 (11%) were randomised within 2 h of symptom onset and another 10 435 (21%) between 2 and 3 h. Fibrinolytic therapy appeared to be beneficial up to at least 12 h (figure 2). The absolute reduction in mortality was greatest among patients who presented within 1 h of symptom onset (average delay 0·75 h). Benefit in this group was estimated at 65 (SD 14; 95% CI 38, 93) lives saved per 1000 treated patients, which is higher than the FTT estimation of benefit at nearly the same time point (0·98 h) of 35 (11). Benefit was also higher in our analysis than in the FTT analysis among patients randomised in the second hour (37 [9]; 20, 55) per 1000 treated. The

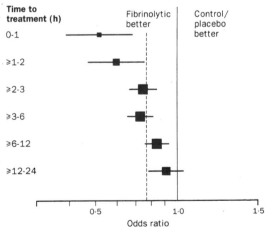

Figure 3: **Proportional effect of fibrinolytic therapy on 35-day mortality according to treatment delay**

Odds ratios, plotted with 95% CI on a log scale, are significantly different over the six groups (Breslow-Day test, p=0·001). Areas of black squares proportional to amount of statistical information

benefit per 1000 treated in the subgroups presenting at ≥2–3 h, ≥3–6 h, ≥6–12 h, and ≥12–24 h was respectively 26 (6; 14, 37), 29 (5; 19, 40), 18 (6; 7, 29), and 9 (7; −5, 22).

Similarly, the proportional mortality reduction was highest in the 1 h patients (48% [95% CI 31, 61]; figure 3), and significantly higher in patients treated within 2 h than in those treated later (44% [32, 53] and 20% [15, 25], respectively). By contrast with the FTT report, odds ratios differed significantly over the time-to-treatment groups (p=0·001, figure 3).

The relation between absolute benefit of fibrinolytic therapy and treatment delay can be described by a linear function, similar to FTT, which shows a significant reduction in benefit of approximately 1·6 (0·5) lives per 1000 patients per hour of treatment delay (H_0: β=0 rejected; p<0·01: R^2=0·22). This linear model was not significantly improved by addition of the term γx² (H_0: γ=0 not rejected; p=0·29; R^2=0·25). However, the component γx⁻¹ of the second non-linear model had a significant contribution to the regression function (H_0: γ=0 rejected; p=0·03). In fact, this latter model fits best with the data (R^2=0·32), in particular with the early observations (figure 4). Inclusion of the USIM and ISIS-3 uncertain indication data and exclusion of the intracoronary studies (WWashICy[26] and ICINy[28]) did not essentially change these findings. Further analyses were performed including all trials with at least 1000 (FTT dataset), 500 and 250 patients, respectively. In all cases, the second non-linear model was significantly better than the linear model.

Discussion

In animals with a coronary circulation similar to that of humans, the amount of myocardial tissue that is salvageable directly depends on the duration of coronary occlusion. This dependency is non-linear. Very early reperfusion of the occluded coronary artery (within 30 min) may lead to full recovery of ischaemic tissue and thus prevent necrosis. In experimental models most of the irreversible damage to the myocardium occurs between 1 and 2 h, after the occlusion, and little or no salvage can be achieved after 6 h of occlusion.

These findings correspond very well with the relation between infarct size estimated by assay of cardiac enzymes and the delay in thrombolytic treatment, as measured in 1334 patients with evolving myocardial infarction.[9] The cumulative release of myocardial α-hydroxybutyrate dehydrogenase during the first 72 h after infarction (Q_{72}) was comparatively small in patients treated within 1 h from onset of symptoms. A very steep increase in the rate of enzyme release was noted between 1 and 2 h of treatment delay (the increase was relatively small thereafter). The life-saving effect of very early reperfusion therapy has been supported by pooled analyses of studies which randomised between immediate, prehospital initiation of therapy and delayed, inhospital therapy (figure 1).[2,22]

This advantage of very early therapy in the prehospital studies is much larger than the effect of 1 h earlier treatment reported by the FTT investigators (1·6 lives per 1000 treated), who compared inhospital thrombolytic with placebo or conventional therapy.[4] We emphasise that patients with a short treatment delay tend to differ from those who wait longer before seeking medical help: many of the patients with very large infarcts (with the highest mortality risk and greatest treatment benefit)[48] report early, whereas elderly patients tend to wait longer.[49,50] Therefore, the randomised comparisons of earlier versus later therapy may provide better estimates of the delay/effect relation than comparison of different cohorts from the large randomised trials. Furthermore, the formal statistical approach has a major influence on the results of the FTT analysis. Results from previous investigations indicating a non-linear delay/benefit relation (eg, the GISSI-1 clinical trial[12]) were considered hypothesis-generating, whereas the outcomes of experimental and prehospital trials were dismissed.[4] In the combined trial data (summarised by five datapoints) no significant deviation of linearity was observed and thus the hypothesis of a linear delay/benefit relation was not rejected in the FTT analysis. By contrast, our alternative analysis supports a non-linear relation which is in agreement with the experimental and prehospital data (figure 4). A large reduction in mortality was detected in patients treated within 1 h of symptom onset (65 [14] per 1000 treated). The decrease in benefit in the 0·75–1·6 h interval (51 min) was roughly 33 lives per 1000 treated per hour (from 65 [14] to 37 [9]), and declined rapidly to about 3·3 lives per h in the 1·6–4·0 h interval (from 37 [9] to 29 [5]), and only 1·4 lives per h after this period (from 29 [5] at 4·0 h to 9 [7] at 18·0 h). The delay/benefit relation could be significantly better described by a non-linear ($\alpha+\beta x+\gamma x^{-1}$) rather than a linear ($\alpha+\beta x$) function. Although the goodness of fit within the tabulated data of the separate trials remains limited (R^2=0·32), the non-linear function does fit very well with the benefit estimations in the six time-to-treatment groups (figure 4).

The concept of a first golden hour in myocardial infarction is supported by our analysis, although our estimations may be biased by differences in baseline characteristics between time-to-treatment groups, the unknown delay between randomisation and actual initiation of therapy and coronary reperfusion, and the unknown individual delays within the reported studies. The benefit of thrombolytic therapy initiated within 30–60 min after onset of symptoms can be estimated at 60–80 additional patients alive at 1 month per 1000 treated compared with conventional therapy. The benefit of therapy within 1–3 h is in the range 30–50 per 1000 treated.

From a clinical standpoint, the challenge is to initiate fibrinolytic treatment within the first 2 to 3 h after symptom onset. A first important step will be to increase public awareness of the need to reduce delay in seeking medical help for cardiac symptoms. Second, as an aid to rapid diagnosis when there is chest pain suggestive of infarction, the general practitioner or ambulance team should obtain—preferably on-site—a computer-interpreted standard 12-lead ECG.[51] With certainty of diagnosis, thrombolytic therapy may be started quickly, before hospital admission. Patients in whom myocardial infarction cannot be confirmed on site, and those presenting directly to the emergency department, may still benefit from emergency room initiation of thrombolytic infusion. Avoidance of unnecessary treatment delay should be given top priority so as to improve the survival prospects of patients with suspected evolving myocardial infarction.[52]

References

1 Vermeer F, Simoons ML, Bär FW, et al. Which patients benefit most from early thrombolytic therapy with intracoronary streptokinase. *Circulation* 1986; 74: 1379–89.

2 Weaver WD. Time to thrombolytic treatment: factors affecting delay and their influence on outcome. *J Am Coll Cardiol* 1995; 25: 3S–9S.

3 Reimer KA, Lowe JE, Rasmussen MM, Jennings RB. The wavefront phenomenon of ischemic cell death: 1 myocardial infarct size versus duration of coronary occlusion in dogs. *Circulation* 1977; 56: 786–94.

4 Fibrinolytic Therapy Trialists' (FTT) Collaborative Group. Indications for fibrinolytic therapy in suspected acute myocardial infarction: collaborative overview of early mortality and major morbidity results from all randomised trials of more than 1000 patients. *Lancet* 1994; 343: 311–22.

5 Flameng W, Lesaffre E, Vanhaecke J. Determinants of infarct size in non-human primates. *Bas Res Cardiol* 1990; 85: 392–403.

6 Reimer KA, Vander Heide RS, Richard VJ. Reperfusion in acute myocardial infarction: effect of timing and modulating factors in experimental models. *Am J Cardiol* 1993; 72: 13G–21G.

7 Dorado DG, Théroux P, Elizaga J, et al. Myocardial infarction in the pig heart model: infarct size and duration of coronary occlusion. *Cardiovasc Res* 1987; 21: 537–44.

8 Schaper W, Binz K, Sass S, Winkler B. Influence of collateral blood flow and of variations in MVO₂ on tissue-ATP content in ischemic and infarcted myocardium. *J Mol Cell Cardiol* 1987; 19: 19–37.

9 Hermens WT, Willems GM, Nijssen KM, Simoons ML. Effect of thrombolytic treatment delay on myocardial infarction size. *Lancet* 1992; 340: 1297.

10 McNeill AJ, Flannery DJ, Wilson CM, et al. Thrombolytic therapy within one hour of the onset of acute myocardial infarction. *Q J Med* 1991; 79: 487–94.

11 Davies GJ, Chierchia S, Maseri A. Prevention of myocardial infarction by very early treatment with intracoronary streptokinase. *N Engl J Med* 1984; 311: 1488–92.

12 Gruppo Italiano per lo Studio della Streptochinasi nell'Infarto miocardico (GISSI). Effectiveness of intravenous thrombolytic treatment in acute myocardial infarction. *Lancet* 1986; i: 397–401.

13 Van de Werf F, Arnold AER, for the European Cooperative Study Group for recombinant tissue type plasminogen activator: intravenous tissue plasminogen activator and size of infarct, left ventricular function, and survival in acute myocardial infarction. *BMJ* 1988; 297: 1374–79.

14 McNeill AJ, Cunningham SR, Flannery DJ, et al. A double-blind placebo-controlled study of early and late adminstration of recombinant tissue plasminogen activator in acute myocardial infarction. *Br Heart J* 1989; 61: 316–21.

15 Schofer J, Büttner J, Geng G, et al. Prehospital thrombolysis in acute myocardial infarction. *Am J Cardiol* 1990; 66: 1429–33.

16 Barbash GI, Roth A, Hod H, et al. Improved survival but not left ventricular function with early and prehospital treatment with tissue plasminogen activator in acute myocardial infarction. *Am J Cardiol* 1990; 66: 261–66.

17 Castaigne AD, Hervé C, Duval-Moulin AM, et al. Pre-hospital use of APSAC: results of a placebo-controlled study. *Am J Cardiol* 1989; 64: 30A–33A.

18 McAleer B, Ruane B, Burke E, et al. Prehospital thrombolysis in a

rural community: short and long-term survival. *Cardiovasc Drugs Ther* 1992; **6:** 369–72.

19 Great Group. Feasibility, safety, and efficacy of domiciliary thrombolysis by general practitioners: Grampian region early anistreplase trial. *BMJ* 1992; **305:** 548–53.

20 Weaver WD, Cerqueira M, Hallstrom AP, et al. Prehospital-initiated vs hospital-initiated thrombolytic therapy: the Myocardial Infarction Triage and Intervention Trial. *JAMA* 1993; **270:** 1211–16.

21 The European Myocardial Infarction Project Group. Prehospital thrombolytic therapy in patients with suspected acute myocardial infarction. *N Engl J Med* 1993; **329:** 383–89.

22 Fath-Ordoubadi F, Al-Mohammad A, Huehns TY, Beat KJ. Meta-analysis of randomised trials of prehospital versus hospital thrombolysis. *Circulation* 1994; **90:** I-325 (abstr).

23 Fath-Ordoubadi F, Beatt KJ. Fibrinolytic therapy in suspected acute myocardial infarction. *Lancet* 1994; **343:** 912.

24 Honan MB, Harrell FE, Reimer KA, et al. Cardiac rupture, mortality and the timing of thrombolytic therapy: a meta-analysis. *J Am Coll Cardiol* 1990; **16:** 359–67.

25 Kennedy JW, Ritchie JL, Davies KB, Fritz JK. Western Washington randomized trial of intracoronary streptokinase in acute myocardial infarction. *N Engl J Med* 1983; **309:** 1477–82.

26 Verstraete M, Bleifeld W, Brower RW, et al. Double-blind randomised trial of intravenous tissue-type plasminogen activator versus placebo in acute myocardial infarction. *Lancet* 1985; ii: 965–99.

27 Simoons ML, Serruys PW, Van den Brand M, et al. Improved survival after early thrombolysis in acute myocardial infarction: a randomised trial by the Interuniversity Cardiology Institute in The Netherlands. *Lancet* 1985; ii: 578–82.

28 Ikram S, Lewis S, Bucknall C, et al. Treatment of acute myocardial infarction with anisoylated plasminogen streptokinase activator complex. *BMJ* 1986; **293:** 786–89.

29 The I.S.A.M. Study Group. A prospective trial of intravenous streptokinase in acute myocardial infarction (I.S.A.M.): mortality, morbidity, and infarct size at 21 days. *N Engl J Med* 1986; **314:** 1465–71.

30 White HD, Norris RM, Brown MA, et al. Effect of intravenous streptokinase on left ventricular function and early survival after acute myocardial infarction. *N Engl J Med* 1987; **317:** 850–55.

31 ISIS-2 (Second International Study of Infarct Survival) Collaborative Group. Randomised trial of intravenous streptokinase, oral aspirin, both, or neither among 17 187 cases of suspected acute myocardial infarction: ISIS-2. *Lancet* 1988; ii: 349–60.

32 AIMS (APSAC Intervention Mortality Study) Trial Study Group. Effects of intravenous APSAC on mortality after acute myocardial infarction: preliminary report of a placebo-controlled clinical trial. *Lancet* 1988; i: 545–49.

33 Wilcox RG, Von der Lippe G, Olsson CG, Jensen G, Skene AM, Hampton JR, for the ASSET Study Group. Trial of tissue plasminogen activator for mortality reduction in acute myocardial infarction. *Lancet* 1988; ii: 525–30.

34 Brunelli C, Spallarossa P, Ghigliotti G, et al. Peaking time of creatine-kinase MB in patients treated with urokinase or conventionally during acute myocardial infarction: is it really a clue to reperfusion? *Cardiologia* 1988; **33:** 669–74.

35 National Heart Foundation of Australia coronary thrombolysis group. Coronary thrombolysis and myocardial salvage by tissue plasminogen activator given up to 4 h after onset of myocardial infarction. *Lancet* 1988; i: 203–07.

36 O'Rourke M, Baron D, Keogh A, et al. Limitation of myocardial infarction by early infusion of recombinant tissue-type plasminogen activator. *Circulation* 1988; **77:** 1311–15.

37 Kennedy JW, Martin GV, David KB, et al. The Western Washington intravenous streptokinase in acute myocardial infarction randomized trial. *Circulation* 1988; **77:** 345–52.

38 Rentrop KP, Feit F, Sherman W, Thornton JC. Serial angiographic assessment of coronary artery obstruction and collateral flow in acute myocardial infarction: report from the second Mount Sinai-New York University reperfusion trial. *Circulation* 1989; **90:** 1166–75.

39 Armstrong PW, Baigrie RS, Daly PA, et al. Tissue plasminogen activator: Toronto (TPAT) placebo-controlled randomized trial in acute myocardial infarction. *J Am Coll Cardiol* 1989; **13:** 1469–76.

40 The Thrombolysis Early in Acute Heart Attack Trial study group. Very early thrombolytic therapy in suspected acute myocardial infarction. *Am J Cardiol* 1990; **65:** 401–07.

41 LATE Study Group. Late Assessment of Thrombolytic Efficacy (LATE) study with alteplase 6–24 h after onset of acute myocardial infarction. *Lancet* 1993; **342:** 759–66.

42 EMERAS (Estudio Multicentrico Esteptoquinasa Republicas de America del Sur) Collaborative Group. Randomised trial of late thrombolysis in patients with suspected acute myocardial infarction. *Lancet* 1993; **342:** 767–72.

43 Rossi P, Bolognese L, on behalf of Urochinasi per la Sistemica nell'Infarto Myocardico (USIM) Collaborative Group. Comparison of intravenous urokinase plus heparin versus heparin alone in acute myocardial infarction. *Am J Cardiol* 1991; **68:** 585–92.

44 ISIS-3 (Third International Study of Infarct Survival) Collaborative Group. ISIS-3: a randomised comparison of streptokinase vs tissue plasminogen activator vs anistreplase and of aspirin plus heparin vs aspirin alone among 41,299 cases of suspected acute myocardial infarction. *Lancet* 1992; **339:** 753–70.

45 Brunelli C, Spallarossa P, Ghigliotta G, Ianetti M, Caponnetto S. Thrombolysis in refractory unstable angina. *Am J Cardiol* 1991; **68:** 110B–18B.

46 Bär FW, Verheugt FW, Col J, et al. Thrombolysis in patients with unstable angina improves the angiographic but not the clinical outcome: results of UNASEM, a multicenter, randomised, placebo-controlled, clincial trial with anistreplase. *Circulation* 1992; **86:** 131–37.

47 The TIMI IIIB investigators. Effects of tissue plasminogen activator and a comparison of early invasive and conservative strategies in unstable angina and non-q-wave myocardial infarction: results of the TIMI IIIB trial. *Circulation* 1994; **89:** 1545–56.

48 Simoons ML, Arnold AER. Tailored thrombolytic therapy. A perspective. *Circulation* 1993; **88:** 2556–64.

49 Turi ZG, Stone PH, Muller JE. Implications for acute intervention related to time of hospital arrival in acute myocardial infarction. *Am J Cardiol* 1986; **58:** 203–09.

50 Yarzebski J, Goldberg RJ, Gore JM, Alpert JS. Temporal trends and factors associated with extent of delay to hospital arrival in patients with acute myocardial infarction: the Worcester heart attack study. *Am Heart J* 1994; **128:** 255–63.

51 Bouten MJM, Simoons ML, Hartman JAM, Van Miltenburg AJM, Van der Does E, Pool J. Prehospital thrombolysis with alteplase (rt-PA) in acute myocardial infarction. *Eur J Heart* 1992; **13:** 925–31.

52 Guidelines. Acute myocardial infarction: pre-hospital and in-hospital management. The task force on the management of acute myocardial infarction of the European society of cardiology. *Eur Heart J* 1996; **17:** 43–63.

Session 4 – Systematic reviews & searching the primary literature

Citation:

Are the results of this systematic review of therapy valid?

Is it a systematic review of randomised trials of the treatment you're interested in?

Does it include a methods section that describes:

• finding and including all the relevant trials?

• assessing their individual validity?

Were the results consistent from study to study?

Are the valid results of this systematic review important?

Translating odds ratios to NNTs. The numbers in the body of the table are the NNTs for the corresponding odds ratios at that particular patient's expected event rate (PEER).

		Odds ratios (OR)								
		0.9	0.85	0.8	0.75	0.7	0.65	0.6	0.55	0.5
	.05	209[1]	139	104	83	69	59	52	46	41[2]
	.10	110	73	54	43	36	31	27	24	21
Control	.20	61	40	30	24	20	17	14	13	11
Event	.30	46	30	22	18	14	12	10	9	8
Rate	.40	40	26	19	15	12	10	9	8	7
(CER)	.50[3]	38	25	18	14	11	9	8	7	6
	.70	44	28	20	16	13	10	9	7	6
	.90	101[4]	64	46	34	27	22	18	15	12[5]

[1] The relative risk reduction (RRR) here is 10%

[2] The RRR here is 49%

[3] For any OR, NNT is lowest when PEER = .50

[4] The RRR here is 1%

[5] The RRR here is 9%

Can you apply this valid, important evidence from a systematic review in caring for your patient?

Do these results apply to your patient?

Is your patient so different from those in the
systematic review that its results can't help you?

How great would the potential benefit of therapy actually be for your individual patient?

Method I: In the table on page 1, find the
intersection of the closest odds ratio from the
systematic review and the CER that is closest to your
patient's expected event rate if they received the
control treatment (PEER):

Method II: To calculate the NNT for any OR and PEER:

$$NNT = \frac{1 - \{PEER \times (1 - OR)\}}{(1 - PEER) \times PEER \times (1 - OR)}$$

Are your patient's values and preferences satisfied by the regimen and its consequences?

Do you and your patient have a clear assessment
of their values and preferences?

Are they met by this regimen and its consequences?

Should you believe apparent qualitative differences in the efficacy of therapy in some subgroups of patients? Only if you can say 'yes' to all of the following:

Do they really make biologic and clinical sense?

Is the qualitative difference both clinically (beneficial
for some but useless or harmful for others) and
statistically significant?

Was this difference hypothesised before the study
began (rather than the product of dredging the
data), and has it been confirmed in other,
independent studies?

Was this one of just a few subgroup analyses carried
out in this study?

Additional notes

Citation: Boersma E, Maas ACP, Deckers JW, *et al*. (1996) Early thrombolytic treatment in acute myocardial infarction: reappraisal of the golden hour. *Lancet*. 348: 771–5.

Are the results of this systematic review of therapy valid?

Is it a systematic review of randomised trials of the treatment you're interested in?	**Yes. They included an analysis of treatment effects *v* time since onset of symptoms.**

Does it include a methods section that describes:

• finding and including all the relevant trials?	**Yes, they captured 22 trials involving over 50,000 patients (but only via MEDLINE)**
• assessing their individual validity?	**Individual trials not well described, so can't tell.**
Were the results consistent from study to study?	**Yes, we think so!**

Are the valid results of this systematic review important?

Translating odds ratios to NNTs. The numbers in the body of the table are the NNTs for the corresponding odds ratios at that particular patient's expected event rate (PEER).

		Odds ratios (OR)								
		0.9	0.85	0.8	0.75	0.7	0.65	0.6	0.55	0.5
	.05	209[1]	139	104	83	69	59	52	46	41[2]
	.10	110	73	54	43	36	31	27	24	21
Control	.20	61	40	30	24	20	17	14	13	11
Event	.30	46	30	22	18	14	12	10	9	8
Rate	.40	40	26	19	15	12	10	9	8	7
(CER)	.50[3]	38	25	18	14	11	9	8	7	6
	.70	44	28	20	16	13	10	9	7	6
	.90	101[4]	64	46	34	27	22	18	15	12[5]

[1] The relative risk reduction (RRR) here is 10%

[2] The RRR here is 49%

[3] For any OR, NNT is lowest when PEER = .50

[4] The RRR here is 1%

[5] The RRR here is 9%

Can you apply this valid, important evidence from a systematic review in caring for your patient?

Do these results apply to your patient?

Is your patient so different from those in the systematic review that its results can't help you?	**Similar, so I can use it.**

How great would the potential benefit of therapy actually be for your individual patient?

Method I: In the table on page 1, find the intersection of the closest odds ratio from the overview and the CER that is closest to your patient's expected event rate if they received the control treatment (PEER):	**Compared with patients treated in hours 2–3, where the NNT to save a life (at 5 weeks) was 27, we need to treat only about half as many (only 15) patients in the first hour to save a life.**

Method II: To calculate the NNT for any OR and PEER:

$$NNT = \frac{1 - \{PEER \times (1 - OR)\}}{(1 - PEER) \times PEER \times (1 - OR)}$$

Are your patient's values and preferences satisfied by the regimen and its consequences?

Do you and your patient have a clear assessment of their values and preferences?	**Would have to be individualised, but benefits far exceed the risks.**
Are they met by this regimen and its consequences?	**Very likely.**

Should you believe apparent qualitative differences in the efficacy of therapy in some subgroups of patients? Only if you can say 'yes' to all of the following:

Do they really make biologic and clinical sense?	**Yes.**
Is the qualitative difference both clinically (beneficial for some but useless or harmful for others) and statistically significant?	**Yes.**
Was this difference hypothesised before the study began (rather than the product of dredging the data), and has it been confirmed in other, independent studies?	**Yes.**
Was this one of just a few subgroup analyses carried out in this study?	**Yes.**

Additional notes

Also see the Fibrinolytic Therapy Trialists' (1994) *Lancet.* 343: 311–22.

MI – GREATER BENEFITS OF THROMBOLYSIS IN THE FIRST HOUR

Appraised by David Sackett 1996.
Expiry date: 1998.

Clinical Bottom Line

In patients requiring thrombolysis for impending myocardial infarction, initiating therapy in the first hour is almost twice as effective (in reducing mortality) as waiting into the second hour.

Citation

Boersma E, Maas ACP, Deckers JW *et al*. (1996) Early thrombolytic treatment in acute myocardial infarction: reappraisal of the golden hour. *Lancet.* **348:** 771–5.

Clinical Question

In a patient with suspected MI, does initiation of thrombolysis within the first hour decrease mortality?

Search Terms

'thrombolysis' and 'myocardial infarction' in *Best Evidence*.

The Study

Systematic review of 22 trials that included 'pain to needle' time.

The Evidence

'Pain to needle' time	0–1 hrs	1–2 hrs	2–3 hrs	3–6 hrs
NNT to save a life at 35 days	15	27	38	34

Comments

See also the Fibrinolytic Therapy Trialists' (1994) *Lancet.* **343:** 311–22.

PART A — Critical appraisal of a systematic review of antihypertensive therapies

In your outpatient clinic you see a 75-year old man with a history of hypertension, who has been on hydrochlorothiazide 25 mg PO OD for 6 months. During this follow-up visit, you note that his blood pressure remains elevated at 180/100 (both arms; no postural drop). He feels well and the remainder of the physical exam is unremarkable.

You wonder whether there is any added benefit to increasing his hydrochlorothiazide or if you should choose an alternate medication. You form the question: 'In an elderly patient with hypertension, do high dose diuretics decrease mortality and stroke compared to low dose diuretics?'

You do a MEDLINE search using the words 'hypertension', 'diuretics', 'mortality' and find a systematic review published in JAMA. You select this article for appraisal. (JAMA (1997) **277**: 739–745)

Read this systematic review and decide:
1 Is this evidence from this systematic review valid?
2 Is this valid evidence from this systematic review important?
3 Can you apply this valid and important evidence from this systematic review when caring for your patient?

If you want to read some strategies for answering these sorts of questions, see pp 97–99, 140–141 and 166–172 in *Evidence-based Medicine*.

EBM SESSION

4

SECTION 2

Systematic reviews & searching the primary literature

PART B Searching for evidence in the primary literature

Colleagues from the library will whet your appetite for learning how to search for evidence in the clinical literature (or hone the searching skills you have already developed), so bring along the clinical questions you generated in Session 2 (or any that you have generated in the meantime). Efficient EBM searching strategies (that trade off the sensitivity and specificity of your searches) are on the next page.

If you haven't already done your search for your presentation in Sessions 6 and 7, now would be a good time to do it!

BEST SINGLE TERMS AND COMBINATIONS FOR HIGH SENSITIVITY MEDLINE SEARCHES ON THE BEST STUDIES OF TREATMENT, DIAGNOSIS, PROGNOSIS, OR CAUSE

Search strategy	Sensitivity[1]	Specificity	Precision
For studies of treatment:			
Clinical trial (pt)	0.93	0.92	0.49
Randomised controlled trial (pt) or Drug therapy (sh) or Therapeutic use (sh) or Random: (tw)	0.99	0.74	0.22
For studies of prognosis:			
Exp cohort studies	0.60	0.80	0.11
Incidence or Exp mortality or Follow up studies or Mortality: (sh) or Prognosis: (tw) or Predict: (tw) or Course: (tw)	0.92	0.73	0.11
For studies of aetiology or cause:			
Risk (tw)	0.67	0.79	0.15
Exp cohort studies or Exp risk or Odds and ratio: (tw) or Relative and risk: (tw) or Case and control: (tw)	0.82	0.70	0.14
For studies of diagnosis:			
Diagnosis (pe)	0.80	0.77	0.09
Exp Sensitivity and specificity or Diagnosis: (pe) or Diagnostic use or Sensitivity: (tw) or Specificity: (tw)	0.92	0.73	0.09

[1] **Sensitivity**, as defined in the study on which the table is based, is the proportion of studies in MEDLINE meeting criteria for scientific soundness and clinical relevance that are detected. **Specificity** is the proportion of less sound/relevant studies that are excluded by the search strategy. **Precision** is the proportion of all citations retrieved that are both sound and relevant. (Source: *Evidence-based Medicine*; also see the Web pages.)

Review

Health Outcomes Associated With Antihypertensive Therapies Used as First-Line Agents

A Systematic Review and Meta-analysis

Bruce M. Psaty, MD, PhD; Nicholas L. Smith, MPH; David S. Siscovick, MD, MPH; Thomas D. Koepsell, MD, MPH; Noel S. Weiss, MD, DrPH; Susan R. Heckbert, MD, PhD; Rozenn N. Lemaitre, PhD, MPH; Edward H. Wagner, MD, MPH; Curt D. Furberg, MD, PhD

Objective.—To review the scientific evidence concerning the safety and efficacy of various antihypertensive therapies used as first-line agents and evaluated in terms of major disease end points.

Data Sources.—MEDLINE searches and previous meta-analyses for 1980 to 1995.

Data Selection.—We selected long-term studies that assessed major disease end points as an outcome. For the meta-analysis, we chose placebo-controlled randomized trials. For randomized trials using surrogate end points such as blood pressure, we selected the largest studies that evaluated multiple drugs. Where clinical trial evidence was lacking, we relied on information from observational studies.

Data Synthesis.—Diuretics and β-blockers have been evaluated in 18 long-term randomized trials. Compared with placebo, β-blocker therapy was effective in preventing stroke (relative risk [RR], 0.71; 95% confidence interval [CI], 0.59-0.86) and congestive heart failure (RR, 0.58; 95% CI, 0.40-0.84). The findings were similar for high-dose diuretic therapy (for stroke, RR, 0.49; 95% CI, 0.39-0.62; and for congestive heart failure, RR, 0.17; 95% CI, 0.07-0.41). Low-dose diuretic therapy prevented not only stroke (RR, 0.66; 95% CI, 0.55-0.78) and congestive heart failure (RR, 0.58; 95% CI, 0.44-0.76) but also coronary disease (RR, 0.72; 95% CI, 0.61-0.85) and total mortality (RR, 0.90; 95% CI, 0.81-0.99). Although calcium channel blockers and angiotensin-converting enzyme (ACE) inhibitors reduce blood pressure in hypertensive patients, the clinical trial evidence in terms of health outcomes is meager. For several short-acting dihydropyridine calcium channel blockers, the available evidence suggests the possibility of harm. Whether the long-acting formulations and the nondihydropyridine calcium channel blockers are safe and prevent major cardiovascular events in patients with hypertension remains untested and therefore unknown.

Conclusion.—Until the results of large long-term clinical trials evaluating the effects of calcium channel blockers and ACE inhibitors on cardiovascular disease incidence are completed, the available scientific evidence provides strong support for the current national guidelines, which recommend diuretics and β-blockers as first-line agents and low-dose therapy for all antihypertensive agents.

JAMA. 1997;277:739-745

From the Cardiovascular Health Research Unit, Departments of Medicine (Drs Psaty, Siscovick, and Koepsell), Epidemiology (Drs Psaty, Smith, Siscovick, Koepsell, Weiss, Heckbert, and Lemaitre), and Health Services (Drs Psaty, Koepsell, and Wagner), University of Washington, and the Center for Health Studies, Group Health Cooperative of Puget Sound (Dr Wagner), Seattle, Wash; and the Department of Public Health Sciences, Bowman Gray School of Medicine, Winston-Salem, NC (Dr Furberg).

Dr Furberg has received research grants from Pfizer and Wyeth-Ayerst and in 1996 received fees for lectures sponsored by Merck and Bristol-Myers Squibb. He also serves on the Data Safety Monitoring Boards for Parke-Davis and Searle. Dr Psaty serves on the Events Committee of a clinical trial funded by Wyeth-Ayerst.

Reprints: Bruce M. Psaty, MD, PhD, Cardiovascular Health Research Unit, Suite 1360, 1730 Minor Ave, Seattle, WA 98101.

IN 1993, the Joint National Committee on the Detection, Evaluation, and Treatment of High Blood Pressure (JNC-V) reversed its previous position about first-line antihypertensive agents.[1] The 1988 JNC-IV guidelines had recommended diuretics, β-blockers, angiotensin-converting enzyme (ACE) inhibitors, and calcium channel blockers as first-line agents.[2] But in 1993, based on the evidence accumulating from long-term clinical trials, the JNC-V characterized low-dose diuretics and β-blockers as "first-choice agents unless they are contraindicated or unacceptable, or unless there are special indications for other agents."[1] Despite these controversial recommendations,[3] ACE inhibitors and calcium channel blockers are widely used as initial drug therapy for hypertension.[4]

With rare exceptions, hypertension is an asymptomatic condition, a risk factor for cardiovascular complications such as stroke, myocardial infarction, and congestive heart failure. The purpose of treatment is to reduce the incidence of these major disease end points. The US Food and Drug Administration approves antihypertensive agents based on their ability to lower blood pressure in short-term trials. But blood pressure lowering in short-term trials may not be a valid surrogate for the outcomes of primary interest with long-term therapy.[5,6] For this reason, the scientific evidence underlying the JNC-V recommendations merits careful attention.

In the present review, we selected studies that evaluated antihypertensive therapies in terms of their ability to prevent stroke and myocardial infarction. We focused on the results of long-term clinical trials, and where clinical trial evidence was lacking, we included information from observational studies. Since the JNC-V encourages the use of the newer agents when "special indications" are present, we also considered the results of the secondary prevention trials in patients with coronary disease or congestive heart failure. We sought to answer the following question: In terms of the scientific evidence regarding health outcomes, which antihypertensive therapies qualify to be used routinely and widely as first-line antihypertensive agents?

METHODS

Using MEDLINE searches and previous meta-analyses,[7-11] we identified studies designed to evaluate the effects of antihypertensive therapies on the occurrence of myocardial infarction and stroke. For randomized trials, the MEDLINE search strategy for 1980 to 1995 was to search based on the terms: (cerebrovascular diseases or heart diseases) and randomized controlled trial and [antihypertensive agents (therapeutic use) or hypertension (drug therapy)]. English and non–English-language abstracts were reviewed. We limited attention to the 4 most commonly used antihypertensive classes (diuretics, β-blockers, calcium channel blockers, and ACE inhibitors).

To be eligible, randomized trials had to be at least 1 year long, placebo controlled, and unconfounded by other therapies. Thus, we excluded multiple risk factor intervention trials,[12,13] trials using first-line agents other than the 4 noted above,[14,15] and trials comparing β-blockers with diuretics.[16,17] No trials evaluating calcium channel blockers or ACE inhibitors were found. All 18 eligible trials,[18-37] which evaluated diuretics or β-blockers, were included in previous meta-analyses,[7-11] and our literature search identified no trial that previous meta-analyses had failed to include. Since the Hypertension Detection and Follow-up Program Study compared a diuretic-based stepped-care therapy with routine community-based referred care (rather than placebo), we listed this trial separately.[21-23] Data were abstracted independently by 2 of us (B.M.P., N.L.S.) and differences were resolved by consensus.

Clinical trials were classified according to the primary treatment strategy used in the active group. While most studies used more than 1 drug in the treated group, the agents were usually applied in a stepped-care approach so that the first-line therapy was clearly identified. The 3 treatment strategies were (1) high-dose diuretic therapy, which used starting doses greater than or equal to the equivalent of 50 mg of chlorthalidone or hydrochlorothiazide[38]; (2) low-dose diuretic therapy, which generally started with the equivalent of 12.5 to 25 mg per day of chlorthalidone or hydrochlorothiazide; and (3) β-blocker therapy. Diuretic dosages were unstated in 2 studies,[29,31] but based on contemporary practice, they were assigned to the high-dose therapy group. The Swedish study[37] was classified as a β-blocker trial since the first-line agent for 68% in the active group was β-blocker therapy.[39]

For ACE inhibitors and calcium channel blockers, we selected the largest and longest trials evaluating surrogate end points. For the special indications, we relied on recent meta-analyses. For observational studies, we sought studies designed to evaluate specific classes of antihypertensive therapies on the occurrence of myocardial infarction or stroke.

In the meta-analysis, we used maximum likelihood methods of combining cumulative incidence risk ratios across the trials, and we examined the data for evidence of heterogeneity.[40] The method of Peto produced nearly identical results.[41] When risk differences were used to estimate the overall effect of therapy in the high-dose diuretic group, the test for homogeneity was rejected for 4 of the 5 outcomes (P<.05). Because the risk difference model did not fit the data well and because previous meta-analyses have generally used risk ratios,[7-11] we present the results in terms of risk ratios. In sensitivity analyses, the results for random-effects models[41] were similar, so we present only the results of the fixed-effects models.

RESULTS

Clinical Trial Evidence Regarding Diuretics and β-Blockers

Taken together, the 18 trials from the United States, Europe, Scandinavia, Australia, and Japan included a total of 48 220 patients followed up for an average of about 5 years. Details about individual trials are provided in previous meta-analyses.[7-11] The high-dose diuretic trials,[18-31] published in the 1970s and 1980s, recruited predominantly middle-aged adults. Some of the small early trials included patients who had very high levels of blood pressure[19] or who had survived a stroke.[28,31] For the low-dose diuretic trials,[32-35] the participants were older adults, sometimes with isolated systolic hypertension,[33,34] and the 2 largest trials were published in the 1990s.[34,35] Several studies evaluated β-blockers as first-line therapy.[26,35-37] The Table summarizes the trial level data.

In the meta-analysis, all 3 treatment strategies reduced the incidence of stroke in patients with hypertension (Figure). The relative risks (RRs) were 0.49, 0.66, and 0.71, and within each treatment-strategy group, there was no statistical evidence of heterogeneity. For stroke prevention, the effect of high-dose diuretic therapy differed from the effect of β-blocker therapy (P=.02) but not from the effect of low-dose diuretic therapy.

For coronary heart disease, the RRs were similar for high-dose diuretic therapy (0.99) and β-blocker therapy (0.93), and neither differed significantly from the placebo. In contrast, low-dose diuretic therapy reduced the incidence of coronary heart disease. The RR of 0.72 differed significantly from the RRs of 0.93 for both β-blocker therapy (P=.03) and of 0.99 for high-dose diuretic therapy (P=.01). There was no statistical evidence of heterogeneity within each of the 3 treatment strategies. In sensitivity analyses, excluding the largest trial or trials with extreme results had trivial effects on these findings.

All 3 treatment strategies were effective in reducing the occurrence of congestive heart failure. Several of the large high-dose diuretic trials[26,35] did not report the incidence of congestive heart failure so that the RR of 0.17 overrepresents the results of early trials that enrolled patients with moderate to severe hypertension.[19,20,28] The reduction in total mortality was significant only for low-dose diuretic therapy (P=.04). For cardiovascular mortality, the reductions were significant for high-dose (P=.03) and low-dose (P<.001) diuretic therapy but not for β-blocker therapy.

In summary, the use of low-dose diuretic therapy, generally in older adults, was associated with important reductions in the incidence of stroke, coronary disease, congestive heart failure, and total mortality. Though evaluated less extensively than diuretics, β-blockers were clearly effective in reducing the incidence of congestive heart failure and stroke in patients with hypertension. Neither β-blocker therapy nor high-dose diuretic therapy was associated with a significant reduction in the incidence of coronary heart disease. Publication bias is an unlikely explanation for this null finding. The RRs of 0.93 to 0.99 differ from the RRs of 0.70 to 0.75 expected on the basis of observational studies.[8,42] Moreover, the slight advantage of β-blockers over high-dose diuretics for coronary disease (0.93 vs 0.99) and the advantage of high-dose diuretic therapy over β-blockers for stroke (0.49 vs 0.71) are consistent with the findings of the large clinical trials that directly compared these 2 therapeutic strategies.[8,16,17,26]

In this analysis, we used the multiplicative model of risk ratios as the summary measure. In the Framingham study, the individual and joint effects of age and high blood pressure on the risk of stroke and coronary disease were well characterized by the multiplicative

Health Outcomes of Antihypertensive Therapies—Psaty et al

Randomized Placebo-Controlled Trials of Antihypertensive Therapy*

Trial†	Rx	Treatment						Control						Duration, y
		CHD	Stroke	CHF	Mortality	CVD	Total	CHD	Stroke	CHF	Mortality	CVD	Total	
VA-NHLBI[18]‡	D-high	8	0	...	2	2	508	5	0	...	0	0	504	1.5
VA-I[19]§	D-high	0	1	0	0	0	73	3	3	4	4	4	70	1.5
VA-II[20]	D-high	11	5	0	10	8	186	13	20	11	21	19	194	3.3
HDFP[21-23]‡||	D-high	171	102	...	349	195	5485	189	158	...	419	240	5455	5.0
Oslo study[24]	D-high	14	0	0	10	7	406	10	5	1	9	6	379	5.5
ANBPS[25]	D-high	33	13	3	25	8	1721	33	22	3	35	18	1706	4.0
MRC[26]‡	D-high	119	18	...	128	69	4297	234	109	...	253	139	8654	4.9
MRC[26]‡	β	103	42	...	120	65	4403	234	109	...	253	139	8654	4.9
USPHS[27]	D-high	15	1	0	2	2	193	18	6	2	4	4	196	7.0
HSCSG[28]¶	D-high	7	37	0	26	15	233	9	42	6	24	19	219	3.0
Barraclough et al[29]#	D-high	1	0	0	1	0	58	2	0	1	3	1	58	2.0
Kuramoto et al[30]**	D-high	1	3	0	7	3	44	2	4	3	7	3	47	4.0
Carter[31]	D-high	2	10	3	13	10	49	2	21	4	22	17	48	4.0
EWPHE[32]	D-low	48	32	19	135	67	416	59	48	23	149	93	424	4.7
Coope and Warrender[36]	β	35	20	22	60	37	419	38	39	36	69	50	465	4.4
MRC-O[35]‡	D-low	48	45	...	134	66	1081	159	134	...	315	180	2213	5.8
MRC-O[35]‡	β	80	56	...	167	95	1102	159	134	...	315	180	2213	5.8
STOP-H[37]	β	25	29	19	36	17	812	28	53	39	63	41	815	2.0
SHEP[34]	D-low	104	103	56	213	90	2365	141	159	109	242	112	2371	4.5
SHEP-P[33]	D-low	15	11	6	32	14	443	4	6	2	7	5	108	2.8

*Rx indicates first-line treatment strategy; CHD, fatal or nonfatal coronary heart disease; CHF, fatal or nonfatal congestive heart failure; CVD, cardiovascular mortality; D-high, high-dose diuretic therapy; D-low, low-dose diuretic therapy; and β, β-blocker therapy. High-dose diuretic therapy included studies that generally used starting drugs and doses greater than or equal to chlorthalidone, 50 mg; hydrochlorothiazide, 50 mg; chlorothiazide, 50 mg; bendroflumethiazide, 5 mg; methyclothiazide, 5 mg; or trichlormethiazide, 2 mg. These dosage equivalences are taken from *Drug Facts and Comparisons, 1996 edition.*[38]

†VA-NHLBI indicates Veterans Administration–National Heart, Lung, and Blood Institute; VA-I, Veterans Administration Cooperative Study Group on Antihypertensive Agents; VA-II, Veterans Administration Cooperative Study Group on Antihypertensive Agents, II; HDFP, Hypertension Detection and Follow-up Program; ANBPS, Australian National Blood Pressure Study; MRC, Medical Research Council; USPHS, US Public Health Service Hospitals; HSCSG, Hypertension-Stroke Cooperative Study Group; EWPHE, European Working Party on High Blood Pressure in the Elderly; MRC-O, Medical Research Council–Older Adults; STOP, Swedish Trial in Old Patients With Hypertension; SHEP, Systolic Hypertension in the Elderly Program; and SHEP-P, Systolic Hypertension in the Elderly Program Pilot Study.

‡No data were available on CHF.

§Data from the original article[19] rather than later analysis.[8]

||CHD includes fatal CHD or nonfatal myocardial infarction by electrocardiograph as reported in the main results[23] and used in a review.[7]

¶Data from original article[28] rather than overview.[8]

#Data were available only for fatal CHF.[29]

**The article did not distinguish between CHF and arrhythmia.[30]

model of risk ratios.[43] The additive model of risk differences did not fit the Framingham data. Similarly, in this meta-analysis, the additive model did not fit the data for high-dose diuretics. When a multiplicative model fits the data well, summary estimates of risk difference depend not only on the effect of the therapy but also on the rate of events in the control group. From the point of view of public health, risk differences are nonetheless an important measure of the effect of interventions. Chatellier and colleagues[44] have developed a nomogram for translating a risk ratio together with the event rate in a population of interest into the clinically useful risk difference measure called "number needed to treat."

Previous meta-analyses of these clinical trials have generally been done in a cumulative fashion.[7-11] While an early meta-analysis[7] had suggested that the treatment of hypertension did not seem to prevent coronary disease, meta-analyses that include more recent trials have tended to conclude that the treatment of hypertension does prevent coronary disease.[8,10,11] This cumulative approach to meta-analysis simply lumps together all 3 treatment strategies as if the effect of blood pressure lowering were independent of the specific antihypertensive drugs and doses used in these trials.

While the 3 treatment regimens lowered blood pressure to a similar degree, the lowering of blood pressure was associated with a reduction in CHD incidence only among subjects randomized to low-dose diuretic therapy. Potential explanations include differences in patient age as well as treatment strategy. The differential effects of the 3 treatment strategies on CHD incidence nonetheless raises questions about the validity of using the lowering of blood pressure as a surrogate end point. Each randomized placebo-controlled clinical trial tests a particular treatment strategy, which includes 1 or more drugs at 1 or more doses, in a population defined by the study's eligibility criteria. Although a study hypothesis may address only the effect of a drug on blood pressure, a large end-point trial evaluating morbidity and mortality is not a test of a single drug effect or mechanism of action. Moreover, trial results are directly generalizable only to that same treatment strategy in other study-eligible patients who, if asked, would have enrolled and participated in a similar trial. Further generalization to other drugs, other doses, or other populations needs to be done cautiously.

Clinical Trial Evidence Regarding Calcium Channel Blockers and ACE Inhibitors

Between 1990 and 1995, 14 525 articles on calcium channel blockers appeared in the MEDLINE literature: 8759 (60.4%) had calcium channel blockers as their primary focus, 1430 (9.8%) were randomized trials, and 1364 (9.4%) were reviews. During the same period, 7256 articles on ACE inhibitors appeared: 5006 (69.0%) had ACE inhibitors as their primary focus, 1144 (15.8%) were randomized trials, and 1210 (16.7%) were reviews. For calcium channel blockers and ACE inhibitors, there were no reports of large, long-term, randomized clinical trials designed to evaluate major disease end points as the primary outcome in hypertensive patients.

Clinical Trials in Hypertension Evaluating Surrogate End Points.—The available trials in hypertension were small short-term studies, and the primary end points were generally metabolic measures, quality of life, levels of blood pressure, or other surrogate end points such

Health Outcomes of Antihypertensive Therapies—Psaty et al **741**

Outcome Drug Regimen	Dose	No. of Trials	Events, Active Treatment/Control	RR (95% CI)	RR (95% CI)
Stroke					
Diuretics	High	9	88/232	0.49 (0.39-0.62)	
Diuretics	Low	4	191/347	0.66 (0.55-0.78)	
β-Blockers		4	147/335	0.71 (0.59-0.86)	
HDFP	High	1	102/158	0.64 (0.50-0.82)	
Coronary Heart Disease					
Diuretics	High	11	211/331	0.99 (0.83-1.18)	
Diuretics	Low	4	215/363	0.72 (0.61-0.85)	
β-Blockers		4	243/459	0.93 (0.80-1.09)	
HDFP	High	1	171/189	0.90 (0.73-1.10)	
Congestive Heart Failure					
Diuretics	High	9	6/35	0.17 (0.07-0.41)	
Diuretics	Low	3	81/134	0.58 (0.44-0.76)	
β-Blockers		2	41/175	0.58 (0.40-0.84)	
Total Mortality					
Diuretics	High	11	224/382	0.88 (0.75-1.03)	
Diuretics	Low	4	514/713	0.90 (0.81-0.99)	
β-Blockers		4	383/700	0.95 (0.84-1.07)	
HDFP	High	1	349/419	0.83 (0.72-0.95)	
Cardiovascular Mortality					
Diuretics	High	11	124/230	0.78 (0.62-0.97)	
Diuretics	Low	4	237/390	0.76 (0.65-0.89)	
β-Blockers		4	214/410	0.89 (0.76-1.05)	
HDFP	High	1	195/240	0.81 (0.67-0.97)	

Meta-analysis of randomized, placebo-controlled clinical trials in hypertension according to first-line treatment strategy. Trials indicate number of trials with at least 1 end point of interest. RR indicates relative risk; CI, confidence interval; and HDFP, Hypertension Detection and Follow-up Program Study (5484 subjects in stepped care and 5455 in referred care). For these comparisons, the numbers of participants randomized to active therapy and placebo were 7768 and 12 075 for high-dose diuretic therapy; 4305 and 5116 for low-dose diuretic therapy; and 6736 and 12 147 for β-blocker therapy. Because the Medical Research Council trials[26] included 2 active arms, the placebo group is included twice in these totals, once for a diuretic comparison and again for a β-blocker comparison. The total number of participants randomized to active therapy and control therapy were 24 294 and 23 926, respectively.

as left ventricular hypertrophy. For example, the recent meta-analysis of reversal of left ventricular hypertrophy[45] identified 39 randomized trials, which included a total of 1394 patients, an average of only 36 patients per study followed for a mean of only 25 weeks.

The Treatment of Mild Hypertension Study (TOMHS) is the largest and the longest of several trials that evaluated multiple therapies.[46,47] In TOMHS, 902 subjects received nutritional hygienic advice and were randomized to placebo or 1 of 5 drug therapies. The blood pressure effects of the 5 drugs were similar over the average follow-up of 4.4 years.[46] All active agents were associated with small reductions in low-density lipoprotein (LDL) cholesterol and glucose as well as small increases in high-density lipoprotein (HDL) cholesterol.[46,48]

While it has been known for years that high-dose diuretic therapy exerts adverse effects on lipids in short-term studies,[49] TOMHS evaluated low-dose diuretic therapy. The average reductions in LDL cholesterol were 0.09 mmol/L (3.6 mg/dL) for placebo, 0.27 mmol/L (10.6 mg/dL) for acebutolol (400 mg/d), 0.13 mmol/L (5.1 mg/dL) for amlodipine maleate (5 mg/d), 0.09 mmol/L (3.6 mg/dL) for chlorthalidone (15 mg/d), 0.29 mmol/L (11.3 mg/dL) for doxazosin mesylate (2 mg/d), and 0.15 mmol/L (5.9 mg/dL) for

enalapril maleate (5 mg/d). Only acebutolol and doxazosin differed significantly from placebo. Compared with low-dose diuretic therapy, the calcium channel blocker and the ACE inhibitor were associated with additional average reductions in LDL cholesterol of only 0.04 mmol/L (1.5 mg/dL) and 0.06 mmol/L (2.3 mg/dL), respectively. These differences in LDL cholesterol were neither statistically nor clinically significant.

The findings of several trials[46,47] suggest that for low-dose diuretic therapy, adverse effects on lipids or glucose tolerance are small or absent and, therefore, not a reason to avoid a proven therapy in patients with hypertension. Whether the lipid advantages of agents such as acebutolol and doxazosin translate into an even greater reduction in the incidence of coronary disease than the 28% reduction achieved by low-dose diuretic therapy (Figure 1) is an important hypothesis, one that remains as yet untested in large clinical trials.

In TOMHS, the combination of 7 quality-of-life indexes indicated significantly greater improvement for participants given chlorthalidone or acebutolol than for those given placebo.[46] For the other 3 drug therapies, the quality-of-life results did not differ from placebo. Similarly, in the Veterans Affairs (VA) trial,[47] patients tolerated hydrochlorothiazide

as well as or better than any of the other 5 drug regimens. The TOMHS data are compatible with the hypothesis that hypertension is a subtly symptomatic condition,[50] one for which treatment with low-dose diuretics and β-blockers improves overall quality of life.

One long-term trial evaluating antihypertensive therapy on carotid wall thickness has reported clinical events as secondary end points.[51] While progression of carotid atherosclerosis was small and similar in both groups, the incidence of major clinical events such as hospitalized angina, myocardial infarction, and stroke was higher in the 442 subjects randomized to isradipine (5-10 mg/d) than in the 441 subjects randomized to hydrochlorothiazide (25-50 mg/d) (RR, 1.78; 95% confidence interval [CI], 0.94-3.38; $P = .07$). In terms of health benefits, the Multicenter Isradipine Diuretic Atherosclerosis Study provides no evidence that this intermediate-acting dihydropyridine is superior to low-dose diuretic therapy.[51]

Clinical Trials of Secondary Prevention.—In terms of health outcomes, the effects of 1 drug used for 1 indication in 1 population may or may not be generalizable to the effects of the same drug for another indication or in another population. A number of critics of the JNC-V recommendations have nonetheless emphasized the "special indications" provision,[3] and they advocate, for instance, the use of ACE inhibitors in hypertensive patients with heart failure and calcium channel blockers in patients with coronary disease.

Calcium Channel Blockers and Coronary Disease.—Among dihydropyridine calcium channel blockers, short-acting nifedipine has been evaluated extensively in clinical trials. In the International Nifedipine Trial on Antiatherosclerotic Therapy trial,[52] nifedipine reduced the occurrence of new coronary lesions at 3 years ($P = .03$), but increased total mortality (12 vs 2 deaths, $P = .008$). Two other nifedipine studies were terminated early when interim analyses suggested the possibility of harm, increased risks of myocardial infarction[53] and early mortality.[54] In a recent meta-analysis,[55] nifedipine, especially in high doses, was associated with an increased risk of mortality. For the 6 trials using 80 mg per day or more of nifedipine, the RR was 2.64 (95% CI, 1.42-4.92). Studies of other short-acting dihydropyridines have also suggested the possibility of harm.[56-59] In short, there is no evidence that short-acting dihydropyridines improve health outcomes in patients with coronary disease.

Many pharmacological properties of the nondihydropyridines such as verapamil and diltiazem differ from the dihydropyridines. Whether these pharmacological differences translate into differences in health outcomes for patients with hypertension remains an untested question. In the setting of established coronary disease, the nondihydropyridines appear to differ from the dihydropyridines.[60,61] Compared with placebo,[61] the nondihydropyridines were associated with reduction in the risk of a second myocardial infarction (RR, 0.79; 95% CI, 0.67-0.94) but not total mortality (RR, 0.95; 95% CI, 0.81-1.10).

ACE Inhibitors and Heart Failure.— Except for early administration in patients with a myocardial infarction,[62] ACE inhibitors have been effective in reducing morbidity and mortality in patients with congestive heart failure.[63] In the meta-analysis by Garg and colleagues,[63] the RR for total mortality was 0.77 (95% CI, 0.67-0.88), and the reduction was primarily due to fewer deaths from progressive heart failure (RR, 0.69; 95% CI, 0.58-0.83). In patients with diabetes, moreover, ACE inhibitors also appear to reduce the incidence of nephropathy,[64] although a recent study in patients with renal failure may suggest the need for caution in the use of benazepril hydrochloride.[65]

In summary, hypertensive patients were generally included in these secondary prevention trials. The results do not provide much support for the use of short-acting dihydropyridines, which are the only dihydropyridine formulations that have been evaluated extensively. In the International Nifedipine Trial on Antiatherosclerotic Therapy,[52] short-acting nifedipine both decreased new coronary lesions and increased total mortality. The most likely explanation lies in the fact that all drugs have multiple effects, and the effects of a drug on a surrogate end point may predict only poorly its effects on major disease end points. Thus, even a well-designed surrogate end point trial may give misleading results from the standpoint of important health outcomes.[5,6]

Based on the health benefits demonstrated in the large clinical trials, several antihypertensive agents clearly have "special indications": (1) ACE inhibitors in patients with congestive heart failure,[63] (2) β-blockers,[66] and (3) nondihydropyridine calcium channel blockers in patients with coronary disease.[61] The evidence for β-blockers is more extensive and compelling than for the nondihydropyridines.[61,66] According to the new guidelines from the American College of Cardiology and the American Heart Association[67]:

[C]alcium-channel blocking agents have not been shown to reduce mortality after acute MI [myocardial infarction], and . . . [it] is the

consensus of this committee that these agents are still used too frequently in patients with acute MI and that beta-adrenoceptor blocking agents are a more appropriate choice across a broad spectrum of patients (with exceptions as noted).[67(p1883)]

Generalization of the results of the secondary prevention trials to all patients with hypertension should be done with caution. Patients with high blood pressure have much lower rates of cardiovascular events than patients with established cardiovascular disease (CVD). Even low rates of adverse events can dramatically alter the overall risk or benefit of a drug therapy. In patients at high risk of cerebrovascular events, for instance, aspirin decreases the occurrence of stroke; but in low-risk populations, the long-term use of aspirin increases the risk of stroke, especially disabling hemorrhagic strokes.[68]

For most of the other "special indications," such as dyslipidemia, renal disease, prostatism, and atrial fibrillation,[3,69] we generally lack information about important health outcomes associated with the "special indication" approach to the choice of drug therapy in patients with high blood pressure. Long-term trials are essential to clarify the risks and benefits of therapies that are used by a variety of high- and low-risk patients for many years.

Evidence From Observational Studies

While the randomized clinical trial is the preferred method of evaluating drug therapies, clinical trial evidence about health outcomes is lacking for commonly used antihypertensive agents. The findings of observational studies can complement those of clinical trials. As noted earlier, the low-dose diuretic trials recruited older adults, and the high-dose diuretic trials included primarily middle-aged adults. Low-dose diuretic therapy, but not the high-dose therapy, was associated with a reduction in the incidence of coronary disease (Figure 1). The clinical trial data alone are unable to address the question of whether this difference in coronary outcomes between high- and low-dose diuretic therapies is the result of diuretic dose or patient age.

Using a case-control design, Siscovick and colleagues[70] reported that, compared with high-dose diuretic therapy, low-dose diuretic therapy with or without a potassium-sparing agent was associated with major reductions in the risk of primary cardiac arrest. With β-blocker users as the reference group, the findings were similar: high-dose thiazides (100 mg/d) were associated with an increased risk (RR, 2.4; 95% CI, 0.7-8.0), but the combination of 25 mg of thiazides and a po-

tassium-sparing agent was associated with a reduced risk of primary cardiac arrest (RR, 0.3; 95% CI, 0.1-1.0). Another case-control study also suggested that the group using mainly potassium-sparing diuretic therapy had a lower risk of sudden cardiac death.[71] Importantly, the associations with diuretic therapy did not differ by patient age. Indeed, the study by Siscovick and colleagues provides strong observational evidence that the dose of the diuretic therapy rather than patient age is responsible for the difference in the effect of diuretic therapies on coronary incidence (Figure).[70]

Observational studies are also important in the postmarketing surveillance of drugs that have been inadequately evaluated in clinical trials. In the Seattle, Wash, case-control study,[72] short-acting calcium channel blockers were associated with an increased risk of myocardial infarction. In the analysis that included only subjects free of CVD, the users of diuretics alone served as the reference group. For subjects taking β-blockers, ACE inhibitors, and calcium channel blockers (with or without diuretics), the adjusted risk ratios were 1.04 (95% CI, 0.74-1.46), 0.89 (95% CI, 0.58-1.38), and 1.62 (95% CI, 1.11-2.34; $P=.01$), respectively. Among subjects with or without CVD, calcium channel blockers were associated with a higher risk of myocardial infarction than β-blockers (risk ratio, 1.57; 95% CI, 1.21-2.04; $P<.001$). Two small case-control studies with limited power failed to confirm these findings.[73,74]

Using data from the Established Populations for Epidemiologic Studies, Pahor and colleagues[75] reported that compared with β-blockers, nifedipine was associated with a 70% increase in mortality (RR, 1.7; 95% CI, 1.1-2.7). The risk of coronary disease was increased in users of diltiazem (RR, 5.0; 95% CI, 2.1-12.3) and nifedipine (RR, 3.5; 95% CI, 1.6-7.8) but not verapamil (RR, 0.7; 95% CI, 0.2-2.4). All calcium channel blockers were associated with an increased risk of heart failure. In contrast, ACE inhibitors were associated with a slightly lower risk of all 3 end points than β-blockers. Several other cohort studies suggest the possibility of higher risks of cardiovascular events in users of nifedipine.[76,77]

Two studies conducted in China and Japan used alternate allocation rather than randomization to assign subjects to treatment or control.[78,79] In the Chinese study,[78] nifedipine in comparison with no therapy was associated with a significant decrease in the risk of stroke. In the Japanese study,[79] cerebrovascular events were more common in subjects on calcium channel blockers than in those on the ACE inhibitor (RR, 2.26; 95% CI, 0.79-6.47). These cohort studies

Session 4 – Systematic reviews & searching the primary literature

do not, however, meet accepted scientific standards for clinical trials.[80] The method of alternate allocation fails to conceal treatment assignment, and the lack of allocation concealment and the lack of double blinding are strongly associated with empirical evidence of bias.[81]

In summary, several large observational studies suggest that short-acting nifedipine may be associated with an increased risk of myocardial infarction and mortality in patients with hypertension. In these studies, ACE inhibitors appear to be comparable to β-blockers and diuretics. Insofar as the findings of observational studies of patients with hypertension are consistent with the findings of clinical trials in patients with other indications for the same therapies, a coherent picture begins to emerge: in terms of health outcomes, both clinical trials and observational studies have identified a problem with the short-acting nifedipine.[82] The recent reports of gastrointestinal bleeding and cancer[83-85] associated with the use of calcium channel blockers have again raised new concerns about a class of agents that have been inadequately evaluated in long-term clinical trials.

Several commentators favor the long-acting dihydropyridine calcium channel blockers since they do not generally produce the sympathetic activation associated with the short-acting formulations.[86,87] This argument, based on a proposed mechanism underlying the adverse effects of the short-acting formulations, is simply another form of the surrogate end point argument. Whether these formulation differences will translate into differences in the incidence of myocardial infarction or stroke in patients with high blood pressure remains an unanswered question. A number of large clinical trials are currently under way or planned,[88,89] but the results will not be available for several years.

COMMENT

Hypertension is a risk factor for major disease end points such as myocardial infarction, congestive heart failure, and stroke. The purpose of therapy is to reduce the incidence of these complications of untreated hypertension. As a result, many patients must receive long-term therapy so that a few may avoid or delay these devastating cardiovascular events. Diuretics and β-blockers—inexpensive antihypertensive agents—have been proven to be both safe and effective in large long-term randomized clinical trials. Recent studies have also given us a new appreciation for the importance of low-dose diuretic therapy for the prevention of coronary disease as well as stroke.

The clinical rationale for withholding safe, effective, and proven therapies must be compelling. For a few subgroups with hypertension, the evidence of health benefits clearly supports the "special indications" approach to choice of therapy: (1) β-blockers in patients with coronary disease; (2) ACE inhibitors in patients with congestive heart failure; and (3) nondihydropyridine calcium channel blockers in patients with coronary disease. We lack clinical trial evidence of major health benefits for most other "special indications." In these situations, the potential benefit in terms of a surrogate end point or a laboratory value must be weighed thoughtfully against the known health risks of withholding the proven first-line therapies currently recommended by the JNC-V.

The research reported in this article was supported by grants HL40628 and HL43201 from the National Heart, Lung, and Blood Institute and AG09556 from the National Institute on Aging. Dr Psaty is a Merck/SER Clinical Epidemiology Fellow sponsored by the Merck Co Foundation, Rahway, NJ, and the Society for Epidemiologic Research, Baltimore, Md.
We appreciate the comments and suggestions from Jeffery Cutler, MD, as well as from anonymous reviewers and editors.

References

1. Joint National Committee on Detection, Evaluation, and Treatment of High Blood Pressure. The Fifth Report of the Joint National Committee on Detection, Evaluation, and Treatment of High Blood Pressure (JNC V). Arch Intern Med. 1993;153:154-183.
2. Joint National Committee on Detection, Evaluation, and Treatment of High Blood Pressure. The 1988 Report of the Joint National Committee on Detection, Evaluation, and Treatment of High Blood Pressure (JNC IV). Arch Intern Med. 1988;148:1023-1038.
3. Tobian L, Brunner HR, Cohn JN, et al. Modern strategies to prevent coronary sequelae and stroke in hypertensive patients differ from the JNC V consensus guidelines. Am J Hypertens. 1994;7:859-872.
4. Manolio TA, Cutler JA, Furberg CD, Psaty BM, Whelton PK, Applegate WB. Trends in pharmacologic management of hypertension in the United States. Arch Intern Med. 1995;155:829-837.
5. Psaty BM, Siscovick DS, Weiss NS, et al. Hypertension and outcomes research: from clinical trials to clinical epidemiology. Am J Hypertens. 1996;9:178-183.
6. Fleming TR, DeMets DL. Surrogate end points in clinical trials: are we being misled? Ann Intern Med. 1996;125:605-613.
7. MacMahon SW, Cutler JA, Furberg CD, Payne GH. The effects of drug treatment for hypertension on morbidity and mortality from cardiovascular disease: a review of randomized controlled trials. Prog Cardiovasc Dis. 1986;29(suppl 1):99-118.
8. Collins R, Peto R, MacMahon S, et al. Blood pressure, stroke, and coronary heart disease, 2: short-term reductions in blood pressure: overview of randomized drug trials in their epidemiologic context. Lancet. 1990;335:827-838.
9. Mulrow CD, Cornell JA, Herrera CR, Kadri A, Farnett L, Aguilar C. Hypertension in the elderly: implications and generalizability of randomized trials. JAMA. 1994;272:1932-1938.
10. Hebert PR, Moser M, Mayer J, Glynn RJ, Hennekens CH. Recent evidence on drug therapy of mild to moderate hypertension and decreased risk of coronary heart disease. Arch Intern Med. 1993;153:578-581.
11. Cutler JA, Psaty BM, MacMahon S, Furberg CD. Public health issues in hypertension control: what has been learned from clinical trials. In: Laragh JH, Brenner BM, eds. Hypertension: Pathophysiology, Diagnosis and Management. 2nd ed. New York, NY: Raven Press; 1995:253-279.
12. Multiple Risk Factor Intervention Trial Research Group. Multiple Risk Factor Intervention Trial: risk factor changes and mortality results. JAMA. 1982;248:1465-1477.
13. Miettinen TA, Huttunen JK, Naukkarinen V, et al. Multifactorial primary prevention of cardiovascular diseases in middle-aged men: risk factor changes, incidence and mortality. JAMA. 1985;254:2097-2102.
14. Wolff FW, Lindeman RD. Effects of treatment in hypertension: results of a controlled study. J Chronic Dis. 1966;19:227-240.
15. Sprackling ME, Mitchell JRA, Short AH, Watt G. Blood pressure reduction in the elderly: a randomised controlled trial of methyldopa. BMJ. 1981;283:1151-1153.
16. The IPPPSH Collaborative Group. Cardiovascular risk and risk factors in a randomized trial of treatment based on the beta-blocker oxprenolol: the International Prospective Primary Prevention Study in Hypertension (IPPPSH). J Hypertens. 1985;3:379-392.
17. Wilhelmsen L, Berglund G, Elmfeldt D, et al. Beta-blockers versus diuretics in hypertensive men: main results from the HAPPHY trial. J Hypertens. 1987;5:561-572.
18. Perry HM Jr, Goldman AI, Lavin MA, et al, for the Veterans Administration-National Heart, Lung, and Blood Institute Group for Evaluating Treatment in Mild Hypertension. Evaluation of drug treatment in mild hypertension: VA-NHLBI feasibility study. Ann N Y Acad Sci. 1978;304:267-288.
19. Veterans Administration Cooperative Study Group on Antihypertensive Agents. Effects of treatment on morbidity in hypertension: results in patients with diastolic blood pressures averaging 115 through 129 mm Hg. JAMA. 1967;202:116-122.
20. Veterans Administration Cooperative Study Group on Antihypertensive Agents. Effects of treatment, II: results in patients with diastolic blood pressure averaging 90 through 114 mm Hg. JAMA. 1970;213:1143-1152.
21. Hypertension Detection and Follow-up Program Cooperative Group. Five-year findings of the Hypertension Detection and Follow-up Program, I: reduction in mortality of persons with high blood pressure, including mild hypertension. JAMA. 1979;242:2562-2571.
22. Hypertension Detection and Follow-up Program Cooperative Group. Five-year findings of the Hypertension Detection and Follow-up Program, III: reduction in stroke incidence among persons with high blood pressure. JAMA. 1982;247:633-638.
23. Hypertension Detection and Follow-up Program Cooperative Group. Effect of stepped care treatment on the incidence of myocardial infarction and angina pectoris: 5-year findings of the Hypertension Detection and Follow-up Program. Hypertension. 1984;6(suppl 1):I198-I206.
24. Hegeland A. Treatment of mild hypertension: a five year controlled drug trial, the Oslo Study. Am J Med. 1980;69:725-732.
25. The Management Committee of the Australian National Blood Pressure Study. The Australian therapeutic trial in mild hypertension. Lancet. 1980;1:1262-1267.
26. Medical Research Council Working Party. MRC trial of treatment of mild hypertension: principal results. BMJ. 1985;291:97-104.
27. Smith WM, for the US Public Health Service Hospitals Cooperative Study Group. Treatment of mild hypertension: results of a ten-year intervention trial. Hypertension. 1977;25(suppl 1):I98-I105.
28. Hypertension-Stroke Cooperative Study Group. Effect of antihypertensive treatment on stroke recurrence. JAMA. 1974;229:409-418.
29. Barraclough M, Joy MD, MacGregor GA, et al. Control of moderately raised blood pressure: report of a co-operative randomized controlled trial. BMJ. 1973;3:434-436.
30. Kuramoto K, Matsushita S, Kuwajima I, Murakami M. Prospective study on the treatment of mild hy-

pertension in the aged. *Jpn Heart J.* 1981;22:75-85.
31. Carter AB. Hypotensive therapy in stroke survivors. *Lancet.* 1970;1:485-489.
32. Amery A, Birkenhager W, Brixko P, et al. Mortality and morbidity from the European Working Party on high blood pressure in the elderly trial. *Lancet.* 1985;1:1350-1354.
33. Perry MH Jr, Smith WM, McDonald RH, et al. Morbidity and mortality in the Systolic Hypertension in the Elderly Program (SHEP) pilot study. *Stroke.* 1989;20:4-13.
34. SHEP Cooperative Research Group. Prevention of stroke by antihypertensive drug treatment in older persons with isolated systolic hypertension: final results of the Systolic Hypertension in the Elderly Program (SHEP). *JAMA.* 1991;265:3255-3264.
35. Medical Research Council Working Party. Medical Research Council trial of treatment of hypertension in older adults: principal results. *BMJ.* 1992; 304:405-412.
36. Coope J, Warrender TS. Randomised trial of treatment of hypertension in elderly patients in primary care. *BMJ.* 1986;243:1145-1151.
37. Dahlof B, Lindholm LH, Hansson L, Schersten B, Ekbom T, Wester PO. Morbidity and mortality in the Swedish Trial in Old Patients With Hypertension (STOP-Hypertension). *Lancet.* 1991;338: 1281-1285.
38. Sewester CS, Dombek CE, Olin BR, Scott JA, Hebel SK, Novak KK, eds. *Drug Facts and Comparisons.* 1996 ed. St Louis, Mo: Facts and Comparisons; 1996.
39. Ekbom T, Dahlof B, Hansson L, Lindholm SH, Schersten B, Wester PO. Antihypertensive efficacy and side effects of three beta-blockers and a diuretic in elderly hypertensives: a report from the STOP-Hypertension study. *J Hypertens.* 1992;10: 1525-1530.
40. Rothman KJ. *Modern Epidemiology.* Boston, Mass: Little Brown & Co Inc; 1986.
41. Berlin JA, Laird NM, Sacks HS, Chalmers TC. A comparison of statistical methods for combining event rates from clinical trials. *Stat Med.* 1989;8: 141-151.
42. MacMahon S, Peto R, Cutler J, et al. Blood pressure, stroke, and coronary heart disease, 1: prolonged differences in blood pressure: prospective observational studies corrected for the regression dilution bias. *Lancet.* 1990;335:765-774.
43. Psaty BM, Koepsell TD, Manolio TA, et al. Risk ratios and risk differences in estimating the effect of risk factors for cardiovascular disease in the elderly. *J Clin Epidemiol.* 1990;43:961-970.
44. Chatellier G, Zapletal E, Lemitre D, Menard J, Degoulet P. The number needed to treat: a clinically useful nomogram in its proper context. *BMJ.* 1996;312:426-429.
45. Schmieder RE, Martus P, Klingbeil A. Reversal of left ventricular hypertrophy in essential hypertension: a meta-analysis of randomized double-blind studies. *JAMA.* 1996;275:1507-1513.
46. Neaton JD, Grimm RH Jr, Prineas RJ, et al, for the Treatment of Mild Hypertension Research Group. Treatment of Mild Hypertension Study (TOMHS): final results. *JAMA.* 1993;270:713-724.
47. Materson BJ, Reda DJ, Cushman WC, et al. Single-drug therapy for hypertension in men: a comparison of six anti-hypertensive agents with placebo. *N Engl J Med.* 1993;328:914-921.
48. Grimm RH Jr, Flack JM, Grandits GA, et al, for the Treatment of Mild Hypertension Study (TOMHS) Research Group. Long-term effects on plasma lipids of diet and drugs to treat hypertension. *JAMA.* 1996;275:1549-1556.
49. Kasiske BL, Ma JZ, Kalil RSN, Louis TA. Effects of antihypertensive therapy on serum lipids. *Ann Intern Med.* 1995;122:133-141.
50. Black HR. Treatment of mild hypertension: the more things change. *JAMA.* 1993;270:757-759.
51. Borhani NO, Mercuri M, Borhani PA, et al. Final outcome results of the Multicenter Isradipine Diuretic Atherosclerosis Study (MIDAS): a randomized controlled trial. *JAMA.* 1996;276:785-791.
52. Lichtlen PR, Hugenholtz PG, Rafflenbeul W, et al. Retardation of angiographic progression of coronary artery disease by nifedipine: results of the International Nifedipine Trial on Antiatherosclerotic Therapy (INTACT). *Lancet.* 1990;335:1109-1113.
53. The HINT Research Group. Early treatment of unstable angina in the coronary care unit: a randomised, double-blind, placebo-controlled comparison of recurrent ischaemia in patients treated with nifedipine or metoprolol or both. *Br Heart J.* 1986; 56:400-413.
54. Goldbourt R, Behar S, Reicher-Reiss H, Zion M, Mandelzweig L, Kaplinsky E, for the SPRINT Study Group. Early administration of nifedipine in suspected acute myocardial infarction: the Secondary Prevention Reinfarction Israel Nifedipine Trial 2 Study. *Arch Intern Med.* 1993;153:345-353.
55. Furberg CD, Psaty BM, Myers JV. Nifedipine: dose-related increase in mortality in patients with coronary heart disease. *Circulation.* 1995;92:1326-1331. Correction: *Circulation.* 1996;93:1475-1476.
56. Thadani U, Sellner SR, Glasser S, et al. Double-blind, dose-response, placebo-controlled multicenter study of nisoldipine: a new second-generation calcium channel blocker in angina pectoris. *Circulation.* 1991;84:2398-2408.
57. Scheidt S, LeWinter MM, Hermanovich J, Venkataraman K, Freedman D. Efficacy and safety of nicardipine for chronic, stable angina pectoris: a multicenter randomized trial. *Am J Cardiol.* 1986; 58:715-721.
58. Gheorghiade M, Weiner DA, Chakko S, Lessem JN, Klein MD. Monotherapy of stable angina with nicardipine hydrochloride: double-blind, placebo-controlled, randomized study. *Eur Heart J.* 1989; 10:695-701.
59. Waters D, Craven TE, Lesperance J. Prognostic significance of progression of coronary atherosclerosis. *Circulation.* 1993;87:1067-1075.
60. Yusuf S, Held P, Furberg C. Update of effects of calcium antagonists in myocardial infarction or angina in light of the second Danish Verapamil Infarction Trial (DAVIT-II) and other recent studies. *Am J Cardiol.* 1991;67:1295-1297.
61. Held PH, Yusuf S. Calcium antagonists in the treatment of ischemic heart disease: myocardial infarction. *Coron Artery Dis.* 1994;5:21-26.
62. Swedberg K, Held P, Kjekshus J, Rasmussen K, Ryden L, Wedel H, on behalf of the CONSENSUS II Study Group. Effects of administration of enalapril on mortality in patients with acute myocardial infarction: results of the Cooperative New Scandinavian Enalapril Survival Study II (CONSENSUS II). *N Engl J Med.* 1992;327:678-684.
63. Garg R, Yusuf S, for the Collaborative Group on ACE Inhibitor Trials. Overview of randomized trials of angiotensin-converting enzyme inhibitors on mortality and morbidity in patients with heart failure. *JAMA.* 1995;273:1450-1456.
64. Viberti G, Mogensen CE, Groop LC, Pauls JF. Effect of captopril on progression to clinical proteinuria in patients with insulin-dependent diabetes mellitus and microalbuminuria. *JAMA.* 1994; 271:275-279.
65. Maschio G, Alberti D, Janin G, et al. Effect of the angiotensin-converting-enzyme inhibitor benazepril on the progression of chronic renal insufficiency. *N Engl J Med.* 1996;334:939-945.
66. Kendall MJ, Lynch KP, Hjalmarson A, Kjekshus J. Beta-blockers and sudden cardiac death. *Ann Intern Med.* 1995;123:358-367.
67. Ryan TJ, Anderson JL, Antman EM, et al. ACC/AHA guidelines for the management of patients with acute myocardial infarction: a report of the American College of Cardiology/American Heart Association Task Force on Practice Guidelines (Committee on Management of Acute MI). *J Am Coll Cardiol.* 1996;28:1328-1428.
68. Antiplatelet Trialists' Collaboration. Collaborative overview of randomised trials of antiplatelet therapy, I: prevention of death, myocardial infarction, and stroke by prolonged antiplatelet therapy in various categories of patients. *BMJ.* 1994;308:81-106.
69. Kaplan NM, Gifford RW Jr. Choice of initial therapy for hypertension. *JAMA.* 1996;275:1577-1580.
70. Siscovick DS, Raghunathan TE, Psaty BM, et al. Diuretic therapy for hypertension and the risk of primary cardiac arrest. *N Engl J Med.* 1994;330: 1852-1857.
71. Hoes AW, Grobbee DE, Lubsen J, Man in 't Veld AJ, van der Does E, Hofman A. Diuretics, beta-blockers, and the risk for sudden cardiac death in hypertensive patients. *Ann Intern Med.* 1995; 123:481-487.
72. Psaty BM, Heckbert SR, Koepsell TD, et al. The risk of myocardial infarction associated with antihypertensive drug therapies. *JAMA.* 1995;274: 620-625.
73. Aursnes I, Litleskare I, Froyland H, Abdelnoor M. Association between various drugs used for hypertension and risk of acute myocardial infarction. *Blood Press.* 1995;4:157-163.
74. Jick H, Derby LE, Guewich V, Vasilakis C. The risk of myocardial infarction associated with antihypertensive drug treatment in persons with uncomplicated essential hypertension. *Pharmacotherapy.* 1996;16:321-326.
75. Pahor M, Guralnik JM, Corti MC, Foley JD, Carbonin P, Havlik RJ. Long-term survival and use of antihypertensive medication in older persons. *J Am Geriatr Soc.* 1995;43:1191-1197.
76. Fallowfield JM, Blenkinsopp J, Raza A, Fowkes AG, Higgins TJ, Bridgman KM. Post-marketing surveillance of lisinopril in general practice in the UK. *Br J Clin Pract.* 1993;47:296-304.
77. Casiglia E, Spolaore P, Mazza A, et al. Effect of two different therapeutic approaches on total and cardiovascular mortality in a Cardiovascular Study in the Elderly (CASTEL). *Jpn Heart J.* 1994;35: 589-600.
78. Gong L, Zwang W, Zhu Y, et al. Shanghai Trial of Nifedipine in the Elderly (STONE) Study. *J Hypertens.* 1996;14:1237-1246.
79. Study Group on Long-term Antihypertensive Therapy. A 12-month comparison of ACE inhibitor and CA antagonist therapy in mild to moderate essential hypertension--the GLANT Study. *Hypertens Res.* 1995;18:235-244.
80. Friedman LM, Furberg CD, DeMets DL. *Fundamentals of Clinical Trials.* 3rd ed. St Louis, Mo: Mosby-Year Book Inc; 1996.
81. Schulz KF, Chalmers I, Hayes RJ, Altman DG. Empirical evidence of bias: dimensions of methodological quality associated with estimates of treatment effects in controlled trials. *JAMA.* 1995;273: 408-412.
82. National Heart, Lung, and Blood Institute. *New Analyses Regarding the Safety of Calcium-Channel Blockers: A Statement for Health Professionals From the National Heart, Lung and Blood Institute.* Bethesda, Md: National Institutes of Health; September 1995.
83. Pahor M, Guralnik JM, Furberg CD, Carbonin P, Havlik RJ. Risk of gastrointestinal haemorrhage with calcium antagonists in hypertensive persons over 67 years old. *Lancet.* 1996;347:1061-1065.
84. Pahor M, Guralnik JM, Salive ME, Corti MC, Carbonin P, Havlik RJ. Do calcium channel blockers increase the risk of cancer? *Am J Hypertens.* 1996;9:695-699.
85. Pahor M, Guralnik JM, Ferrucci L, et al. Calcium channel blockers and incidence of cancer in aged populations. *Lancet.* 1996;348:493-497.
86. Epstein M. Calcium antagonists should continue to be used as first-line treatment of hypertension. *Arch Intern Med.* 1995;155:2150-2156.
87. Lindqvist M, Kahan T, Melcher A, Hjemdahl P. Acute and chronic calcium antagonist treatment elevates sympathetic activity in primary hypertension. *Hypertension.* 1994;24:287-296.
88. Davis BR, Cutler JA, Gordon DJ, et al, for the ALLHAT Research Group. Rationale and design for the Antihypertensive and Lipid Lowering Treatment to Prevent Heart Attack Trial (ALLHAT). *Am J Hypertens.* 1996;9:342-360.
89. Slovick DK, Amery A, Birkenhager W, et al. SYST-EUR multicentre trial on the treatment of isolated systolic hypertension in the elderly: first interim report. *J Hum Hypertens.* 1993;7:201-203.

Citation:

Are the results of this systematic review of therapy valid?

Is it a systematic review of randomised trials of the treatment you're interested in?

Does it include a methods section that describes:

• finding and including all the relevant trials?

• assessing their individual validity?

Were the results consistent from study to study?

Are the valid results of this systematic review important?

Translating odds ratios to NNTs. The numbers in the body of the table are the NNTs for the corresponding odds ratios at that particular patient's expected event rate (PEER).

		Odds ratios (OR)								
		0.9	0.85	0.8	0.75	0.7	0.65	0.6	0.55	0.5
	.05	209[1]	139	104	83	69	59	52	46	41[2]
	.10	110	73	54	43	36	31	27	24	21
Control	.20	61	40	30	24	20	17	14	13	11
Event	.30	46	30	22	18	14	12	10	9	8
Rate	.40	40	26	19	15	12	10	9	8	7
(CER)	.50[3]	38	25	18	14	11	9	8	7	6
	.70	44	28	20	16	13	10	9	7	6
	.90	101[4]	64	46	34	27	22	18	15	12[5]

[1] The relative risk reduction (RRR) here is 10%

[2] The RRR here is 49%

[3] For any OR, NNT is lowest when PEER = .50

[4] The RRR here is 1%

[5] The RRR here is 9%

Can you apply this valid, important evidence from a systematic review in caring for your patient?

Do these results apply to your patient?

Is your patient so different from those in the
systematic review that its results can't help you?

How great would the potential benefit of therapy actually be for your individual patient?

Method I: In the table on page 1, find the
intersection of the closest odds ratio from the
systematic review and the CER that is closest to your
patient's expected event rate if they received the
control treatment (PEER):

Method II: To calculate the NNT for any OR and PEER:

$$NNT = \frac{1 - \{PEER \times (1 - OR)\}}{(1 - PEER) \times PEER \times (1 - OR)}$$

Are your patient's values and preferences satisfied by the regimen and its consequences?

Do you and your patient have a clear assessment
of their values and preferences?

Are they met by this regimen and its consequences?

Should you believe apparent qualitative differences in the efficacy of therapy in some subgroups of patients? Only if you can say 'yes' to all of the following:

Do they really make biologic and clinical sense?

Is the qualitative difference both clinically (beneficial
for some but useless or harmful for others) and
statistically significant?

Was this difference hypothesised before the study
began (rather than the product of dredging the
data), and has it been confirmed in other,
independent studies?

Was this one of just a few subgroup analyses carried
out in this study?

Additional notes

Citation: Psaty BM, Smith NL, Siscovick DS *et al.* (1997) Health outcomes associated with antihypertensive therapies used as first-line agents. *JAMA.* 277: 739–45.

Are the results of this systematic review of therapy valid?

Is it a systematic review of randomised trials of the treatment you're interested in?	**Yes.**
Does it include a methods section that describes: • finding and including all the relevant trials?	**Yes. Identified studies using MEDLINE and previous systematic reviews – English and non-English abstracts reviewed.**
• assessing their individual validity?	**Does not describe if studies evaluated for validity but does explain some differences in inclusion criteria in various studies.**
Were the results consistent from study to study?	**Yes – no heterogeneity.**

Are the valid results of this systematic review important?

Translating odds ratios to NNTs. The numbers in the body of the table are the NNTs for the corresponding odds ratios at that particular patient's expected event rate (PEER).

					Odds ratios (OR)					
		0.9	0.85	0.8	0.75	0.7	0.65	0.6	0.55	0.5
	.05	209[1]	139	104	83	69	59	52	46	41[2]
	.10	110	73	54	43	36	31	27	24	21
Control	.20	61	40	30	24	20	17	14	13	11
Event	.30	46	30	22	18	14	12	10	9	8
Rate	.40	40	26	19	15	12	10	9	8	7
(CER)	.50[3]	38	25	18	14	11	9	8	7	6
	.70	44	28	20	16	13	10	9	7	6
	.90	101[4]	64	46	34	27	22	18	15	12[5]

[1] The relative risk reduction (RRR) here is 10%

[2] The RRR here is 49%

[3] For any OR, NNT is lowest when PEER = .50

[4] The RRR here is 1%

[5] The RRR here is 9%

Can you apply this valid, important evidence from a systematic review in caring for your patient?

Do these results apply to your patient?

Is your patient so different from those in the overview that its results can't help you?	**Sufficiently similar to be helpful.**

How great would the potential benefit of therapy actually be for your individual patient?

Method I: In the table on page 1, find the intersection of the closest odds ratio from the overview and the CER that is closest to your patient's expected event rate if they received the control treatment (PEER):	**total mortality:** *high dose diuretics* **– PEER = 0.139, RRR = 12%, then ARR is 0.139 x .12 = 0.017 and the NNT is 59 (but need to look at confidence interval)** *low dose diuretics* **– PEER = 0.139, RRR = 10%, then ARR is 0.139 x .10 = .0139 and the NNT is 72**

Method II: To calculate the NNT for any OR and PEER:

$$NNT = \frac{1 - \{PEER \times (1 - OR)\}}{(1 - PEER) \times PEER \times (1 - OR)}$$

Are your patient's values and preferences satisfied by the regimen and its consequences?

Do your patient and you have a clear assessment of their values and preferences?	**Needs to be assessed in each patient.**
Are they met by this regimen and its consequences?	**Needs to be assessed in each patient.**

Should you believe apparent qualitative differences in the efficacy of therapy in some subgroups of patients? Only if you can say 'yes' to all of the following:

Do they really make biologic and clinical sense?	**Yes.**
Is the qualitative difference both clinically (beneficial for some but useless or harmful for others) and statistically significant?	**Yes.**
Was this difference hypothesised before the study began (rather than the product of dredging the data), and has it been confirmed in other, independent studies?	**Yes.**
Was this one of just a few subgroup analyses carried out in this study?	**Yes.**

Additional notes

None.

Clinical Bottom Line
Low and high dose diuretics decrease total mortality and stroke.

Citation
Psaty BM, Smith NL, Siscovick DS *et al.* (1997) Health outcomes associated with antihypertensive therapies used as first-line agents. *JAMA* **277**: 739–45.

Clinical Question
In an elderly patient with hypertension, do high dose diuretics decrease mortality and stroke compared to low dose diuretics?

Search Terms
'hypertension', 'stroke' and 'mortality' in *Best Evidence.*

The Study
Systematic review of 18 RCTs with a total of 48 220 patients. Follow up an average of 5 yrs.

The Evidence

Stroke:

Medication	PEER	RRR (CI)	ARR (CI)	NNT (CI)
High dose diuretics:				
• high risk patients	.068	.51 (.38 to .61)	.035 (.026 to .041)	29 (24 to 39)
• low risk patients	.019	.51 (.38 to .61)	.010 (.007 to .012)	100 (83 to 142)
Low dose diuretics:				
• high risk patients	.068	.34 (.23 to .45)	.023 (.016 to .031)	43 (33 to 63)
• low risk patients	.019	.34 (.23 to .45)	.007 (.004 to .009)	143 (111 to 250)

Total Mortality:

Medication	PEER	RRR (CI)	ARR (CI)	NNT (CI)
High dose diuretics:				
• high risk patients	.139	.12 (−.03 to .25)	.017 (−.004 to .035)	59 (NNH 250 to NNT 29)
• low risk patients	.032	.12 (−.03 to .25)	.064 (−.001 to .008)	250 (NNH 1000 to NNT 125)
Low dose diuretics:				
• high risk patients	.139	.1 (.01 to .19)	.014 (.001 to .026)	72 (38 to 1000)
• low risk patients	.032	1 (.01 to .19)	.003 (.0003 to .006)	333 (167 to 3333)

HYPERTENSION – DIURETICS DECREASE TOTAL MORTALITY

Appraised by Sharon Straus.
Expiry date: 1998.

Comments

1 High dose diuretic trials recruited predominantly middle-aged adults and these pts are termed low risk in the above table

2 Low dose diuretic trials recruited older subjects and these pts are called high risk in the above table

3 Need information about side-effects that occur with high v low dose diuretics which is not available from this article

Session 4 – Systematic reviews & searching the primary literature

PART A — Critical appraisal of a clinical article about harm

You see a 73-year old man in your general medicine clinic who has a history of hypertension for which he has been taking nifedipine XL 30 mg PO per day for five years. In his retirement he has learned how to use the Internet and he brings you a print-out of some newspaper headlines that he unearthed while surfing the net:

'Hypertension Med Kills'
LA Times

'Drug for blood pressure linked to heart attacks: researchers fear 6 million are imperilled'
Washington Post

He is very worried and wants to know if he should stop taking nifedipine. Together, you form the clinical question: 'In patients taking calcium antagonists for hypertension, do these calcium antagonists cause cancer? You track down the *Lancet* article referred to in the scary newspaper article (*Lancet* (1996) **348:** 493-7).

Read this article and decide:
1 Are the results of this harm study valid?
2 Are the results of this harm study important?
3 Should these valid, important results of this study about a potentially harmful treatment change the treatment of your patient?

If you want to read some strategies for answering these sorts of question, see pp 105–10, 147–9 and 179–81 in *Evidence-based Medicine*.

PART B — Searching for evidence on the WWW

We will show you how to access the Web and introduce you to the web page for the Centre for Evidence-Based Medicine in Oxford (http://cebm.jr2.ox.ac.uk/), where there are data banks of clinically useful measures on the precision and accuracy of clinical exam and lab test results (SpPins, SnNouts, sensitivities, specificities, likelihood ratios), the power of prognostic factors and therapy (NNTs, RRRs and the like), plus the CATMaker and links to several other centres and sources of evidence.

To help us organize your presentations for Sessions 6 and 7, please complete and hand in the form on the next page.

CASE PRESENTATION

My tentative clinical question:

My name: _____

Contact address: _____

Contact phone number: _____

Bleep: _____

E-mail: _____

Session 5 – Harm & surfing the Web for evidence

Articles

Calcium-channel blockade and incidence of cancer in aged populations

Marco Pahor, Jack M Guralnik, Luigi Ferrucci, Maria-Chiara Corti, Marcel E Salive, James R Cerhan, Robert B Wallace, Richard J Havlik

Summary

Background Calcium-channel blockers can alter apoptosis, a mechanism for destruction of cancer cells. We examined whether the long-term use of calcium-channel blockers is associated with an increased risk of cancer.

Methods Between 1988 and 1992 we carried out a prospective cohort study of 5052 people aged 71 years or more and who lived in three regions of Massachusetts, Iowa, and Connecticut USA. Those taking calcium-channel blockers (n=451) were compared with all other participants (n=4601). The incidence of cancer was assessed by survey of hospital discharge diagnoses and causes of death. These outcomes were validated by the cancer registry in the one region where it was available. Demographic variables, disability, cigarette smoking, alcohol consumption, blood pressure, body-mass index, use of other drugs, hospital admissions for other causes, and comorbidity were all assessed as possible confounding factors.

Findings The hazard ratio for cancer associated with calcium-channel blockers (1549 person-years, 47 events) compared with those not taking calcium-channel blockers (17 225 person-years, 373 events) was 1·72 (95% CI 1·27–2·34, p=0·0005), after adjustment for confounding factors. A significant dose-response gradient was found. Hazard ratios associated with verapamil, diltiazem, and nifedipine did not differ significantly from each other. The results remained unchanged in community-specific analyses. The association between calcium-channel blockers and cancer was found with most of the common cancers.

Interpretation Calcium-channel blockers were associated with a general increased risk of cancer in the study populations, which suggested a common mechanism. These observational findings should be confirmed by other studies.

Lancet 1996; **348:** 493–97

See Editorial page 487

See Commentary pages 488 and 489

Introduction

Calcium-channel blockers are prescribed primarily for

Department of Internal Medicine and Geriatrics, Catholic University, Rome, Italy (M Pahor MD); **Epidemiology, Demography, and Biometry Program, National Institute on Aging, Bethesda, MD, USA** (J M Guralnik MD, M-C Corti MD, M E Salive MD, R J Havlik MD); **Geriatric Department, I Fraticini, Istituto Nazionale Ricerca e Cura Per Gli Anziani (INRCA), Florence, Italy** (L Ferrucci MD); **and Department of Preventive Medicine and Environmental Health, University of Iowa, IA, USA** (J R Cerhan MD, R B Wallace MD)

Correspondence to: Dr Marco Pahor, Department of Preventive Medicine, University of Tennessee, Memphis, 66 N Pauline, Suite 232, Memphis, TN 38105, USA

treatment of hypertension and coronary heart disease but lately their long-term safety has been questioned.[1-4] Excess all-cause mortality has been associated with the use of short-acting nifedipine.[1,2] Calcium-channel blockers are potent drugs that affect various organ systems. Calcium-channel blockers are used to treat oesophageal diseases,[5] and cause constipation,[6] increase risk of haemorrhage,[7,8] and can impair differentiation during embryogenesis.[9] Furthermore, cases of lupus after use of diltiazem have been reported.[10]

We have hypothesised that calcium-channel blockers increase the risk of cancer by interfering with physiological mechanisms that regulate cancer cell growth.[4,11] Evidence is emerging that calcium-channel blockers can block apoptosis,[12-14] an efficient mechanism for limiting cancer growth.[15-18] Calcium-channel blockers might affect cancer risk generally or be limited to specific sites where calcium mechanisms predominate. For example, colon cancer has been related to reduced calcium ingestion.[19]

In this prospective study, the initial analyses done in individuals receiving treatment for hypertension[11] have been extended to the general older population. The aim was to assess whether individuals taking calcium-channel blockers, for any indication were at higher risk of developing cancer than those not taking those drugs. The study focused on specific cancers, additional potential confounding factors, and the effects of dose.

Methods

The study was based on the Established Populations for Epidemiologic Studies of the Elderly (EPESE)—a collaborative, prospective cohort study of older persons supported by the US National Institute on Aging.[20] The participants surveyed were from three regions. Between 1982 and 1983, a regional survey was carried out on all persons aged 65 years or older living in East Boston, Massachusetts, and in the counties of Iowa and Washington in the state of Iowa. During the same period of time another survey was done in New Haven, Connecticut, where a random sample stratified by housing type and sex was taken.

Over 80% of the eligible population was interviewed. At the initial EPESE interview, and after 3 and 6 years of follow-up, trained interviewers administered a 90-min questionnaire that covered a wide range of psychosocial and health-related issues. Telephone follow-up interviews were done 1, 2, 4, and 5 years after the initial interview. Cancer events were assessed for the time between the sixth EPESE annual follow-up in 1988 and the end of 1992.

Information on date of hospital admission and up to five discharge diagnoses for each person in the survey was gathered from the Health Care Financing Administration Medicare Provider Analysis and Review (MEDPAR) files. The match of EPESE participants with MEDPAR files was complete from Jan 1, 1985, until Dec 31, 1992.

Vital status on Dec 31, 1992, was assessed at the seventh follow-up (Iowa and Connecticut) by contact with relatives, examination of obituaries in local newspapers, and linkage with the National Death Index.[21] One nosologist studied death certificates and then used ICD-9 codes to record the underlying, immediate, and contributing causes of death. Hospital discharge diagnoses or causes of death with ICD-9 codes 140–208 recorded at any time in the MEDPAR files were defined as cancer events. Specific codes were used to identify site of cancer.

In previous studies, hospital chart reviews provided validation of cancer as a hospital discharge diagnosis.[22] In this study, in the individuals from the Iowa regions cancer outcomes were validated by matching of the EPESE participants with the State Health Registry of Iowa's cancer registry, which is part of the National Cancer Institute's Surveillance, Epidemiology, and End Results (SEER) program.[23] The kappa statistic[24] for the agreement of the MEDPAR files and death certificates with the SEER registry in ascertaining prevalent (before baseline), incident, and any prevalent or incident cancer cases was 0·77, 0·83, and 0·86, respectively.

During the section of the baseline interview on the use of medications, participants were asked to show all containers for all prescription and non-prescription drugs taken over the past 2 weeks. The interviewer transcribed the drug product name from the container label. If the label was not seen, the interviewer asked the participant the name of the drug. These ascertainment methods are similar to those of other studies and have proven valid and reliable.[25,26] Participants taking calcium-channel blockers were compared with participants who were not. In addition, separate analyses were done for verapamil, nifedipine, and diltiazem.

For participants living in Massachussetts and Iowa the daily dose of calcium-channel blocker was calculated; the strength of the drug product was multiplied by the number of times the medication was taken per day. In Connecticut the dose could not be calculated. The median dose was established for verapamil, nifedipine, and diltiazem separately (240, 30, and 180 mg/day, respectively), then the calcium-channel blocker dose was ranked as low (below median), median, or high (over median).

The following factors potentially associated with cancer were assessed at the baseline interview: age; sex; ethnic origin; coronary heart disease (use of nitrates, self-report of heart attack, any hospital discharge diagnosis coded 410–414 in the preceding 3 years, or a positive Rose questionnaire for angina assessed at any interview giving in person[27]); heart failure (use of both digoxin and a diuretic, or any hospital discharge diagnosis coded 428 in the preceding 3 years); hypertension (systolic blood pressure ≥140 mm Hg or diastolic ≥90 mm Hg measured at any visit, self-report of a medical diagnosis of hypertension, or any hospital discharge diagnosis coded 401 in the preceding 3 years); stroke (self-report of stroke, or any hospital discharge diagnosis coded 430–434 in the preceding 3 years); diabetes (use of antidiabetic drugs, self-report of diabetes, or any hospital discharge diagnosis coded 250 in the preceding 3 years); use of β-blockers, angiotensin-converting enzyme (ACE) inhibitors, diuretics, digoxin, nitrates, non-steroidal anti-inflammatory drugs, aspirin, corticosteroids, oestrogens, or coumarin; current smoking status (non-smoker or smoking 1–19 or ≥20 cigarettes per day); alcohol intake (≥28·35 g/day, assessed by self-reported frequency and number of consumed drinks of beer, wine, and spirits); and physical disability (limitation in one or more of the following: walking half a mile, climbing a flight of stairs, doing heavy housework, walking across a room, bathing, dressing, eating, or transferring from bed to chair).[28,29] Trained interviewers measured blood pressure two or three times according to the Hypertension Detection and Follow-up Program protocol.[30] The mean of the last two measurements was calculated. Body-mass index was calculated from reported weight and height. The number of hospital admissions before the qualifying event or before the end of follow-up was assessed.

Of the original population of more than 10 000 interviewed in 1982, 6566 participants were still alive and were interviewed in 1988, the baseline period for this study. We excluded 298 participants who could not be matched with MEDPAR files, and 1216 participants who reported a cancer at any of the interviews, who had a hospital discharge diagnosis of cancer in the 3 years

Characteristic	Not taking calcium-channel blockers (n=4601)	Taking calcium-channel blockers (n=451)	p*
Demographic			
Mean (SE) age	79·3 (0·1)	79·0 (0·3)	p>0·1
Women	64·5%	64·1%	p>0·1
Ethic origin			
White	94·2%	93·6%	
Black	5·1%	6·4%	p>0·1
Other	0·7%	0	
Comorbid conditions			
Coronary heart disease	21·9%	71·2%	p<0·0001
Heart failure	9·7%	29·3%	p<0·0001
Hypertension	81·7%	90·0%	p<0·0001
Stroke	9·2%	12·6%	p=0·016
Diabetes	15·7%	26·2%	p<0·0001
Medications			
β-blockers	11·6%	23·3%	p<0·0001
ACE inhibitors	4·4%	8·6%	p<0·0001
Diuretics	33·5%	50·6%	p<0·0001
Digoxin	11·6%	25·1%	p<0·0001
Nitrates	6·2%	38·8%	p<0·0001
NSAIDs	12·5%	14·6%	p>0·1
Aspirin	29·7%	37·3%	p<0·001
Oestrogens	0·8%	0·2%	p>0·1
Corticosteroids	3·2%	3·8%	p>0·1
Coumarin	2·6%	6·0%	p<0·0001
Mean (SE) blood pressure (mm Hg)			
Systolic	136 (0·4)	138 (1·3)	p>0·1
Diastolic	73 (0·2)	72 (0·6)	p=0·033
Mean (SE) body-mass index (kg/m²)	24·4 (0·1)	24·8 (0·3) ·	p>0·1
Smoking status			
Current non-smoker	90·1%	91·8%	p>0·1
1–19 cigarettes per day	4·9%	5·3%	
≥20 cigarettes per day	3·8%	2·7%	
Alcohol intake ≥28·35 g per day	5·0%	4·4%	p>0·1
Health indicators			
Physical disability	45·4%	62·7%	p<0·0001
Mean (SE) number of hospital admissions	1·2 (0)	2·2 (0·1)	p<0·0001

Percentages may not total 100% because of missing data. *χ² test for categorical variables, ANOVA or Mann-Whitney tests for comparison of means. ACE=angiotensin converting enzyme. NSAIDs=non-steroidal anti-inflammatory drugs.

Table 1: **Population baseline characteristics according to use of calcium-channel blockers**

before the study baseline, or who were taking anticancer drugs such as tamoxifen. The remaining population at risk was 5052 participants (1741 from East Boston, 2020 from Iowa, and 1291 from New Haven).

The first cancer event that occurred during follow-up was used as a primary endpoint. Participants with no events, by the time of the final follow-up in 1992 were censored on Dec 31, 1992, or at the time of death, whichever occurred first. The Kaplan-Meier method was used to plot survival free of cancer. Cox proportional hazards regression models were used to estimate the hazard ratio and 95% CI for the association of variables of interest with cancer. The assumption of proportionality of hazard was assessed with log minus log plots and by tests of the interaction of exposure with time. In multivariate models, additional indicator variables were created to adjust for the effects of missing data for cigarette smoking, alcohol intake, and disability (1·1%, 0·8%, and 6·8% with missing data, respectively). In analyses summarising results for all three regions, the regression models were stratified by region.

Results

Compared with participants who were not taking calcium-channel blockers those taking these drugs were significantly more likely to have cardiovascular diseases and diabetes, to use cardiovascular drugs, to be disabled, to have a lower diastolic blood pressure, and to be

494

Session 5 – Harm & surfing the Web for evidence

	Number of events	Person-years	Rate per 1000 person-years	Unadjusted model		Adjusted model*	
				Hazard ratio (95% CI)	p	Hazard ratio (95% CI)	p
All calcium-channel blockers							
Non-users (n=4601)	373	17 225	21·7	1	..	1	..
Users (n=451)	47	1549	30·3	1·42 (1·05–1·92)	0·032	1·72 (1·27–2·34)	0·0005
Individual calcium-channel blockers							
Verapamil (n=118)	18	420	42·9	2·03 (1·26–3·25)	0·0035	2·49 (1·54–4·01)	0·0002
Nifedipine (n=146)	16	480	33·3	1·56 (0·94–2·51)	0·083	1·74 (1·05–2·88)	0·031
Diltiazem (n=184)	13	641	20·3	0·94 (0·54–1·63)	>0·1	1·22 (0·70–2·12)	>0·1

*Adjusted for age, sex, ethnic origin, heart failure, number of hospital admissions, cigarette smoking, and alcohol intake. Three participants were excluded from the analyses of individual calcium-channel blockers because they were taking two calcium-channel blockers.

Table 2: **Use of calcium-channel blockers and their relation to cancer**

admitted to hospital (table 1). Age, sex, ethnic origin, cigarette smoking, alcohol intake, systolic blood pressure, body-mass index, and use of non-cardiovascular drugs did not differ significantly between the two groups.

During 18 774 person-years of follow-up (mean follow-up time 3·7 years), 420 participants had a cancer event (140 in East Boston, 185 in Iowa, and 95 in New Haven; overall rate 22·4 per 1000 person-years; table 2). The most frequent cancers were those of the colon, prostate, lung, lymphatic and haemopoietic organs, urinary tract, and breast (table 3). 169 people died from cancer (9·0 per 1000 person-years).

Users of calcium-channel blockers had significantly higher crude rates of cancer than non-users (table 2, figure 1). Patients taking verapamil had the highest rate of cancer followed by patients taking nifedipine and diltiazem.

To assess independent risk factors for cancer that might have confounded the association of calcium-channel blockers with cancer, separate proportional hazard regression models (adjusted for age and sex) were calculated for groups of variables, including demographic characteristics, chronic diseases, medications, and general health indicators (cigarette smoking, alcohol intake, physical disability, blood pressure, body-mass index, and number of hospital admissions). In the initial models there were significant associations between age, being male, being black, cigarette smoking, and alcohol consumption and increased risk of cancer. An inverse relation with cancer was found for heart failure and number of hospital admissions (p<0·1). In a summary multivariate model adjusted for these potential confounding factors, calcium-channel blocker users had a

significantly increased risk of cancer compared with all other participants (hazard ratio=1·72, p=0·0005, table 2). The association was significant for verapamil and nifedipine, but not for diltiazem. However, the difference in hazard ratio among specific calcium-channel blockers was not significant. In the fully adjusted models the hazard ratios were greater than those calculated without adjustment. In separate models adjusted for confounding factors and either systolic and diastolic blood pressure or any past diagnosis of hypertension, the hazard ratio of cancer associated with calcium-channel blockers was 1·67 (1·21–2·29), and 1·71 (1·25–2·32), respectively. The hazard ratio associated with use of β-blockers, ACE inhibitors, diuretics, digoxin, nitrates, non-steroidal anti-inflammatory drugs, aspirin, corticosteroids, or coumarin was not significant and was close to 1 (not shown).

In community-specific multivariate analyses, the hazard ratio of cancer for calcium-channel blocker users was 1·55 (0·89–2·71), 1·82 (1·12–2·98), and 1·84 (1·04–3·26), compared with all other participants, in East Boston, Iowa, and New Haven, respectively. Daily dose of calcium-channel blocker was assessed in East Boston and Iowa and increasing dose was associated with a significant gradient of increased hazard ratio of cancer when compared with those who did not use calcium-channel blockers (figure 2).

Separate multivariate models stratified according to potential risk factors of cancer were calculated. The hazard ratio of cancer for calcium-channel blockers was 1·77 (1·20–2·63) in participants aged 71–79 years (n=2982) and 1·55 (0·93–2·59) in those aged 80 years and older (n=2070); 1·64 (1·09–2·46) in men (n=1796) and 1·81 (1·13–2·90) in women (n=3256); 1·60 (1·15–2·22) in white people (n=4757) and 3·42 (1·25–9·39) in black people (n=264); 1·78 (1·29–2·47) in those not currently cigarette smokers (n=4559) and 1·44 (0·55–3·73) in current cigarette smokers (n=439); 1·76 (1·27–2·42) in those drinking <28·35 g of alcohol per day (n=4762) and 1·26 (0·42–3·73) in those drinking ≥28·35 g of alcohol per day (n=252); 1·71 (1·23–2·37) in those with any lifetime diagnosis of hypertension (n=4163) and 1·99 (0·78–5·07) in those with no hypertension (n=889); 1·80 (1·17–2·76) in those with diastolic and systolic blood pressure below 90 mm Hg and below 140 mm Hg, respectively (n=2313); and 1·57 (0·97–2·54) in those with elevated (≥90/140 mm Hg) blood pressure (n=1969).

In multivariate models stratified by number of hospital admissions, and in analyses that excluded cancer events in which a circulatory disease (ICD 9 codes 390–459) was the principal discharge diagnosis, the results for calcium-channel blockers were unchanged (summary hazard ratio for the stratified models 1·70 [1·25–2·31], and 1·62, [1·18–2·24], respectively). When individual cancer sites were analysed separately, calcium-channel blocker use

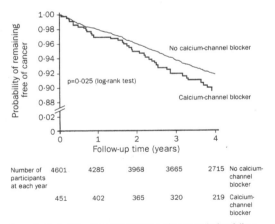

Figure 1: **Probability of remaining free of cancer during follow-up according to use of calcium-channel blockers**

Session 5 – Harm & surfing the Web for evidence

Type of cancer (ICD-9 code)	Number of events	Hazard ratio (95% CI)
Stomach (151)	13	3·64 (0·96–13·76)
Colon (153)	65	1·98 (0·90–4·38)
Rectum (154)	23	1·32 (0·31–5·74)
Liver, gallbladder, pancreas (155–157)	24	1·15 (0·26–4·96)
Lung (162)	56	0·21 (0·03–1·52)
Skin (172–173)	14	1·11 (0·14–8·62)
Breast (174)	31	1·65 (0·49–5·55)*
Uterus, adnexa (182–183)	23	3·69 (1·22–11·14)*
Prostate (185)	58	1·99 (0·93–4·27)
Bladder, ureter, kidney (188–189)	38	1·57 (0·55–4·47)
Lymphatic, haemopoietic (200–208)	46	2·57 (1·13–5·83)

Regression models stratified by community and adjusted for age, sex, ethnic origin, heart failure, number of hospital admissions, cigarette smoking, and alcohol intake.
*Adjusted for oestrogen use.

Table 3: **Relation of use of calcium-channel blockers with specific types of cancer**

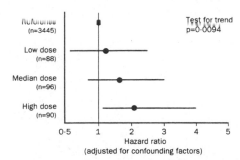

Figure 2: **Hazard ratio and 95% CI of incident cancer according to daily dose of calcium-channel blocker compared with no calcium-channel blocker use**
Estimates are adjusted for age, sex, ethnic origin, heart failure, number of hospital admissions, smoking, and alcohol intake. Median daily dose for verapamil, nifedipine, and diltiazem 240, 30, and 180 mg.

was associated with a significantly increased hazard ratio for cancers of the uterus and adnexa uteri, and lymphatic and haemopoietic organs (table 3). The hazard ratio was increased, but did not reach significance for stomach, colon, rectum, breast, prostate, and urinary tract cancers. For liver, gallbladder and pancreas, and skin cancers, the hazard ratio was increased, but close to 1. A non-significant inverse relation was found for lung cancer (table 3).

Separate analyses used the Iowa SEER cancer registry data rather than the MEDPAR files or death certificates to define the population that was free of cancer at baseline and incident cases of cancer. In these analyses, the incidence rate of cancer was 12·1 per 1000 person-years among participants not taking calcium-channel blockers (120 events, 1829 participants) and 30·4 per 1000 person-years among those taking calcium-channel blockers (16 events, 106 participants, p<0·001). After adjustment for confounding factors, the hazard ratio of cancer associated with calcium-channel blocker use was 3·09 (1·80–5·31), p<0·0001.

Discussion

We found that after adjustment for confounding factors, older people taking calcium-channel blockers for any indication had a significant 70% excess hazard ratio of developing cancer during 3·7 years (mean) of follow-up compared with those not taking these drugs. This association was consistent in all three regions in this study, and for most types of cancer. The dose-response gradient was significant. The excess risk of cancer associated with use of calcium-channel blockers was even more evident when the SEER cancer registry information was used to define the events. No association with cancer was found for other cardiovascular medications.

If calcium-channel blockers truly promote cancer, what are the potential mechanisms? Apoptosis, or programmed cell death, is an efficient physiological mechanism for elimination of cells with genetic lesions, and, therefore, for preventing cancer.[15] Calcium-channel blockers inhibit apoptosis in various experimental models by interfering with calcium-triggered signals.[12,14,18] At therapeutic concentrations, verapamil and nifedipine suppress gene activity associated with involution by apoptosis of prostate and breast after the removal of physiological hormone stimulation.[12,31] Such mechanisms may also prevent apoptosis of neoplastic cells, thereby promoting cancer growth.[11] Inhibition of calcium-mediated cell differentiation may also play a part.[18]

The consistent association of calcium-channel blockers with increase in most types of cancer found in this study suggests that calcium-channel blockers might promote cancer through a common underlying biological process, such as interference with apoptosis or cell differentiation. Calcium-channel blockers may act as cancer promoters but standard carcinogenicity bioassays, which are designed to identify chemical mutagens, may fail to recognise such promoters. Further research is needed to assess whether the inverse relation of calcium-channel blockers with lung cancer was produced by chance alone or by other specific mechanisms.

Calcium-channel blocker use was ascertained at baseline and the latent period required for producing a clinically relevant cancer could not be calculated. Interestingly the Kaplan-Meier curves start diverging at about 2 years after the start of the study. The latent period for the underlying mechanism by which calcium-channel blockers might promote cancer may be less than that needed for chemical mutagens.

Calcium-channel blockers can potentiate anticancer drugs and facilitate apoptosis. However, such effects were observed in animal and in-vitro models at toxic concentrations not tolerated in man, and were accompanied by a paradoxical increase in intracellular calcium.[32]

We have identified six potential limitations of the study. First, although several confounding factors were examined, observational data such as these cannot conclusively establish causal links. Whether calcium-channel blockers truly promote cancer needs to be confirmed in long-term clinical trials. Physical disabilities and the consequent incapacity of a number of participants in this study would probably preclude their attendance for follow-up visits. Thus, these individuals would probably be excluded from clinical trials.

Second, users of calcium-channel blockers had higher rates than the non-users of hospital admission for cardiovascular disease; this difference could have led to a bias in cancer detection. However, the significant calcium-channel blocker cancer association did not change after adjustment or stratification on number of hospital admissions, and after exclusion of cancer hospital admissions in which a circulatory disease was the principal diagnosis. Use of other antihypertensive agents, nitrates, digoxin, corticosteroids, and anticoagulants, which are used for treating diseases requiring frequent medical surveillance, was not associated with cancer.

Patients with heart failure, who are frequently admitted to hospital, tended to have a lower hazard ratio of cancer. Patients who are elderly and have an important cardiovascular condition might not undergo cancer screening as often as those who are healthy.

A third possible limitation was that exposure and outcome may have been misclassified. Drug use was assessed only at baseline and some participants may have stopped taking calcium-channel blockers during follow-up. Furthermore, cancers that did not lead to hospital admission or death were not ascertained, and the diagnoses in the MEDPAR files and death certificates may not be accurate. However, such potential misclassifications would probably dilute any associations found and introduce a conservative bias, leading to an underestimation of the association of calcium-channel blocker use with cancer.

Fourth, our findings in older people who have higher rates of cancer may not be applicable to younger individuals. Fifth, mainly short-acting calcium-channel blockers were used in this study. Theoretically, with new calcium-channel blockers and the slow-release formulations the plasma concentrations may remain below a harmful threshold. Finally, hypertension has been associated with an increased risk of cancer mortality in middle-aged people.[33,34] However, in this study blood pressure was not related to cancer and did not confound the calcium-channel blocker-cancer association.

Evaluation of long-term safety and efficacy of medications such as calcium-channel blockers, which exert multiple and incompletely identified actions, needs to focus on assessment of major outcomes and survival.[1-3,8,35,36] A judgment about the clinical implications of our findings is currently premature. The evidence provided by this single study is not sufficient to recommend withdrawal of treatment from current users. However, these observational data should stimulate further experimental, epidemiological, and clinical research to assess all the cardiovascular and non-cardiovascular effects of calcium-channel blockers.

This study was supported by contracts N01-AG-0-2105, N01-AG-0-2106, and N01-AG-0-2107 from the National Institute on Aging, Bethesda, MD, USA. MP was supported by a grant from Ministero per l'Università e Ricerca Scientifica e Tecnologica, 60% N7020532, and from Consiglio Nazionale delle Ricerche, Italy, N95000959PF40.

References

1 Pahor M, Guralnik JM, Corti C, Foley DJ, Carbonin PU, Havlik RJ. Long-term survival and use of antihypertensive medications in older persons. *J Am Geriatr Soc* 1995; 43: 1191–97.

2 Furberg CD, Psaty BM, Meyer JV. Nifedipine. Dose-related increase in mortality in patients with coronary heart disease. *Circulation* 1995; 92: 1326–31.

3 Psaty BM, Heckbert SR, Koepsell TD, et al. The risk of myocardial infarction associated with antihypertensive drug therapies. *JAMA* 1995; 274: 620–25.

4 Furberg CD, Pahor M, Psaty BM. The unnecessary controversy. *Eur Heart J* 1996; 17: 1142–47.

5 Konrad Dalhoff I, Baunack AR, Ramsch KD, et al. Effect of the calcium antagonists nifedipine, nitrendipine, nimodipine and nisoldipine on oesophageal motility in man. *Eur J Clin Pharmacol* 1991; 41: 313–16.

6 Pahor M, Guralnik JM, Chrischilles EA, Wallace RB. Use of laxative medication in older persons and associations with low serum albumin. *J Am Geriatr Soc* 1994; 42: 50–56.

7 Wagenknecht LE, Furberg CD, Hammon JW, Legault C, Troost BT. Surgical bleeding: unexpected effect of a calcium antagonist. *BMJ* 1995; 310: 776–77.

8 Pahor M, Guralnik JM, Furberg CD, Carbonin PU, Havlik RJ. Risk of gastrointestinal haemorrhage with calcium antagonists in hypertensive persons over 67 years old. *Lancet* 1996; 347: 1061–65.

9 Stein G, Srivastava MK, Merker HJ, Neubert D. Effects of calcium channel blockers on the development of early rat postimplantation embryos in culture. *Arch Toxicol* 1990; 64: 623–38.

10 Crowson AN, Magro CM. Diltiazem and subacute cutaneous lupus erythematosus-like lesions. *N Engl J Med* 1995; 333: 1429.

11 Pahor M, Guralnik JM, Salive ME, Corti MC, Carbonin P, Havlik RJ. Do calcium channel blockers increase the risk of cancer? *Am J Hypertens* 1996; 9: 695–99.

12 Connor J, Sawczuk IS, Benson MC, et al. Calcium channel antagonists delay regression of androgen-dependent tissues and suppress gene activity associated with cell death. *Prostate* 1988; 13: 119–30.

13 Juntti Berggren L, Larsson O, Rorsman P, et al. Increased activity of L-type Ca^{2+} channels exposed to serum from patients with type I diabetes. *Science* 1993; 261: 86–90.

14 Ray SD, Kamendulis LM, Gurule MW, Yorkin RD, Corcoran GB. Ca^{2+} antagonists inhibit DNA fragmentation and toxic cell death induced by acetaminophen. *FASEB J* 1993; 7: 453–63.

15 Carson DA, Ribeiro JM. Apoptosis and disease. *Lancet* 1993; 341: 1251–54.

16 Trump BF, Berezesky IK. Calcium-mediated cell injury and cell death. *FASEB J* 1995; 9: 219–28.

17 Martin SJ, Green DR. Apoptosis and cancer: the failure of controls on cell death and cell survival. *Crit Rev Oncol Hematol* 1995; 18: 137–53.

18 Whitfield JF. Calcium signals and cancer. *Crit Rev Oncog* 1992; 3: 55–90.

19 Garland C, Shekelle RB, Barrett-Connor E, Criqui MH, Rossof AH, Paul O. Dietary vitamin D and calcium and risk of colorectal cancer: a 19-year prospective study in men. *Lancet* 1985; i: 307–09.

20 Cornoni-Huntley J, Ostfeld AM, Taylor JO, et al. Established populations for epidemic studies of the elderly: study design and methodology. *Aging Clin Exp Res* 1993; 5: 27–37.

21 Stampfer MJ, Willett WC, Speizer FE, Dysert DC. Test of the National Death Index. *Am J Epidemiol* 1984; 119: 837–39.

22 Fisher ES, Whaley FS, Krushat WM, et al. The accuracy of Medicare's hospital claims data: progress has been made, but problems remain. *Am J Public Hlth* 1992; 82: 243–48.

23 SEER cancer statistics review, 1973–1991: tables and graphs, National Cancer Institute. NIH publication No 94-2789. Bethesda, MD: NIH publication no 94-2789, 1994.

24 Cohen J. Weighted kappa: nominal scale agreement with provision for scaled disagreement or partial credit. *Psychol Bull* 1968; 70: 213–20.

25 Psaty BM, Lee M, Savage PJ, Rutan GH, German PS, Lyles M. Assessing the use of medications in the elderly: methods and initial experience in the Cardiovascular Health Study. *J Clin Epidemiol* 1992; 45: 638–92.

26 Pahor M, Chrischilles EA, Guralnik JM, Brown SL, Wallace RB, Carbonin PU. Drug data coding and analysis in epidemiologic studies. *Eur J Epidemiol* 1994; 10: 405–11.

27 Rose GA, Blackburn H, Gillum RF, Prineas RJ. Annex 6—London school of hygiene cardiovascular questionnaire. In: World Health Organisaton. Cardiovascular survey methods, 2nd edn. Geneva: WHO, 1982: 162–65.

28 Katz S, Ford AB, Moskowitz RW, Jackson BA, Jaffe MW. Studies of illness in the aged. The index of ADL: a standardized measure of biological and psychosocial function. *JAMA* 1963; 185: 94–99.

29 Rosow I, Breslau N. A Guttman health scale for the aged. *J Gerontol* 1966; 21: 556–59.

30 Hypertension Detection and Follow-up Program Cooperative Group. Blood pressure studies in 14 communities; a two-stage screen for hypertension. *JAMA* 1977; 237: 2385–91.

31 Tenniswood MP, Guenette RS, Lakins J, Mooibroek M, Wong P, Welsh JE. Active cell death in hormone-dependent tissues. *Cancer Metastasis Rev* 1992; 11: 197–220.

32 Batra S, Popper LD, Hartley-Asp B. Effect of calcium and calcium antagonists on 45Ca influx and cellular growth of human prostatic tumor cells. *Prostate* 1991; 19: 299–311.

33 Raynor WJ, Shekelle RB, Rossof AH, Maliza M, Paul O. High blood pressure and 17-year cancer mortality in the Western Electric Health Study. *Am J Epidemiol* 1981; 118: 371–77.

34 Dyer AR, Stamler J, Berkson DM, Lindberg HA, Stevens E. High blood pressure: a risk factor for cancer mortality? *Lancet* 1975; i: 1051–56.

35 Furberg CD, Psaty BM. Calcium antagonists: antagonists or protagonists of mortality in elderly hypertensives? *J Am Geriatr Soc* 1995; 43: 1309–10.

36 Yusuf S. Calcium antagonists in cornary artery disease and hypertension. Time for reevaluation? *Circulation* 1995; 92: 1079–82.

Citation:

Are the results of this harm study valid?

Were there clearly defined groups of patients, similar in all important ways other than exposure to the treatment or other cause?

Were treatment exposures and clinical outcomes measured the same way in both groups, e.g. was the assessment of outcomes either objective (death) or blinded to exposure?

Was the follow up of study patients complete and long enough?

Do the results satisfy some 'diagnostic tests for causation'?

- Is it clear that the exposure preceded the onset of the outcome?

- Is there a dose-response gradient?

- Is there positive evidence from a 'dechallenge-rechallenge' study?

- Is the association consistent from study to study?

- Does the association make biological sense?

Are the valid results from this harm study important?

		Adverse outcome		Totals
		Present (case)	Absent (control)	
Exposed to the Treatment	Yes (cohort)	a	b	a+b
	No (cohort)	c	d	c+d
	Totals	a+c	b+d	a+b+c+d

In a randomised trial or cohort study: relative risk = RR = [a/(a+b)]/[c/(c+d)]
In a case-control study: odds ratio (or Relative odds) = OR = ad/bc
In this study:

Should these valid, potentially important results of a critical appraisal about a harmful treatment change the treatment of your patient?

Can the study results be extrapolated to your patient?

What are your patient's risks of the adverse outcome?
To calculate the NNH[1] for any odds ratio (OR) and your patient's expected event rate for this adverse event if they were **not** exposed to this treatment (PEER):

$$NNH = \frac{PEER\,(OR - 1) + 1}{PEER\,(OR - 1) \times (1 - PEER)}$$

What are your patient's preferences, concerns and expectations from this treatment?

What alternative treatments are available?

Additional notes

[1] The number of patients you need to treat to harm one of them.

Citation: Pahor M *et al.* (1996) Calcium-channel blockade and incidence of cancer in aged populations. *Lancet.* **348**: 493–97 (see also pp 487–9 and 541–2).

Are the results of this harm study valid?

Were there clearly defined groups of patients, similar in all important ways other than exposure to the treatment or other cause?	**Clearly defined but heterogeneous. Exposed individuals different from non-exposed – more diabetes and cardiovascular disease, disability, hospitalization but lower diastolic pressure – but both groups cancer-free at the start of the study.**
Were treatment exposures and clinical outcomes measured the same way in both groups, e.g. was the assessment of outcomes either objective (death) or blinded to exposure?	**Yes. Asked to show their medications and clinical outcomes measured the same way in both groups.**
Was the follow up of study patients complete and long enough?	**Averaged 3.7 years and long enough to show a positive relationship between CCBs and cancer. But there were only 47 cancers in 1549 person-years of CCB taking.**

Do the results satisfy some 'diagnostic tests for causation'?

• Is it clear that the exposure preceded the onset of the outcome?	**Probably – excluded everyone with known cancer at the start (still may have been some smouldering).**
• Is there a dose-response gradient?	**Yes – Figure 2.**
• Is there positive evidence from a 'dechallenge-rechallenge' study?	**No**
• Is the association consistent from study to study?	**No**
• Does the association make biological sense?	**Whether interference with apoptotic destruction of cancer cells is sensible is hotly debated.**

BUT: was this a previously generated hypothesis, or was it one of several analyses carried out on a large data set of drugs and diseases? (We have written to the authors about this and Dr Pahor has informed us that this hypotheses was generated prior to the study onset.)

Are the valid results from this harm study important?

		Adverse outcome		Totals
		Present (case)	Absent (control)	
Exposed to the Treatment	Yes (cohort)	3.03% a	b	a+b
	No (cohort)	c 2.17%	d	c+d
	Totals	a+c	b+d	a+b+c+d

In this study: relative risk = RR = 3.03%/2.17% = 1.4 (P = 0.032) (and when adjusted for several baseline differences, RR ROSE (!) to 1.7 (P = 0.0005)).

Should these valid, potentially important results of a critical appraisal about a harmful treatment change the treatment of your patient?

Can the study results be extrapolated to your patient?	**Depends on whether you believe them. If you do believe them, they can be extrapolated to your patient.**
What are your patient's risks of the adverse outcome? To calculate the NNH[1] for any odds ratio (OR) and your patient's expected event rate for this adverse event if they were **not** exposed to this treatment (PEER): NNH = $\dfrac{\text{PEER (OR} - 1) + 1}{\text{PEER (OR} - 1) \times (1 - \text{PEER})}$	**If we assume our patient is like the average individual in this study (the hazard ratios are like odds ratios and don't differ in important ways between subgroups), then his absolute risk increase in cancer over 3.7 years is 3.03% - 2.17% = 0.86% = and 1/0.86% gives an NNH of 116.**
What are your patient's preferences, concerns and expectations from this treatment?	**Need to be determined.**
What alternative treatments are available?	**Lots of alternative treatments available for his hypertension (thiazides, beta-blockers). They have their own side-effects but are not reputed to cause cancer.**

Additional notes

1   Other case-control and cohort studies vary in their conclusions about CCB risks and a meta-analysis is awaited.

Until it is sorted out, you could describe NNTs (and possible NNHs) for alternative antihypertensive regimens with your patient and the two of you could collaborate in deciding on the most appropriate one for him.

[1] The number of patients you need to treat to harm one of them.

HYPERTENSION – CALCIUM-CHANNEL BLOCKERS MAY CAUSE CANCER

Appraised by David Sackett 1996.
Expiry date: 1998.

Clinical Bottom Line

1 Until this gets sorted out properly, if your patient's problem could be treated as well by some alternative drug, e.g. hypertension, it would be prudent to avoid using calcium-channel agents.

2 If this result is true, the NNH to cause one additional cancer from taking CCBs for 3.7 years is 116.

Citation

Pahor M *et al*. (1996) Calcium-channel blockade and incidence of cancer in aged populations. *Lancet*. **348:** 493–97 (see also pp 487–9 and 541–2).

Clinical Question

In patients taking calcium antagonists for hypertension, are they at increased risk of cancer?

Search Terms

From the newspaper headline or from MEDLINE using 'calcium antagonists' and 'cancer'.

The Study

Total or stratified random samples (>80% response rate) of 65+ year old men and women in three sites in the USA. They showed their meds, were interviewed for 90 minutes and had their blood pressure, height and weight measured. Anyone with cancer in the previous three years or on any cancer Rx was excluded and 94% of the remainder were followed for an average of 3.7 years by follow-up interview, hospital discharge information and the national death registry for the occurrence of new cancers.

The Evidence

		Later cancer		Totals
		Present	Absent	
Exposed to calcium Channel blockers	Yes (cohort)	3.03% a	b	a+b
	No (cohort)	2.17% c	d	c+d
	Totals	a+c	b+d	a+b+c+d

Relative risk = RR = 3.03%/2.17% = 1.4 (P = 0.032) (and when adjusted for several baseline differences, RR ROSE (!) to 1.7 (P = 0.0005)).

Comments

1 Individuals on CCBs had more cardiovascular disease, diabetes, disability and hospitalizations but lower diastolic blood pressure. But when they adjusted for all these baseline differences, the RR rose

rather than fell, suggesting that bias from confounding (of cancer risk and CCB use) of these characteristics could not explain these results.

2   There was a dose-response gradient.

3   The difference in risk by type of CCB was impressive but not statistically significant (RR 2 for verapamil; 1.5 for nifedipine; 0.94 for diltiazem).

4   Only 47 events in CCB takers and spread over all sorts of different cancers.

5   The proposed mechanism (interference with the apoptotic destruction of cancer cells) dismissed by commentators.

6   Other studies of CCBs and mortality go both ways (they are bad or have no effect), and some authors of the former have received anonymous death threats.

NOTES ON THE INTERNET

The Internet: why bother?
- Networking with colleagues.
- Getting hold of useful documents for free.
- Publishing useful information for free.
- Bypassing traditional publishers and online vendors.

EBM on the Internet
- e-mail discussion list (run by Mailbase):
  evidence-based-health@mailbase.ac.uk

To join send an e-mail to **mailbase@mailbase.ac.uk** with an empty subject field and the following as the only text of the message itself: **join evidence-based-health Joe Bloggs**

To get list of mailbase discussion lists, send this command in the same way to the same address: **find lists medical**

To get a mailbase user guide, send the command: **send mailbase user-guide**

- The EBM Toolbox (the CEBM World-Wide Web site)
  http://cebm.jr2.ox.ac.uk/

See links to other sites (especially SCHARR) in Other Resources. It also has:
- a glossary of EBHC terms and research methodologies
- how to focus a clinical question
- educational prescriptions
- hints on how to optimise MEDLINE searches
- detailed definitions and examples of NNTs, SpPINs and SnNOUTs, likelihood ratios, pre-test probabilities, prognostic indicators
- scenarios used in the teaching packs at our workshops
- worksheets for critical appraisal.

Searching for stuff on the Web
- Use other people's links to good sites. An excellent place to start for this is the Netting the Evidence and SCHARR Project at Sheffield: **http://panizzi.shef.ac.uk/auracle/links.html**
- To find your own good sites, use the search engines, such as:

Altavista:	**www.altavista.com**
Excite:	**www.excite.com**
Lycos:	**www.lycos.com**
Yahoo!:	**www.yahoo.com**

There is a good site with links to all the best internet search engines at: **http://alt.venus.co.uk/weed/search/welcome.htm**
- The browser's **Find** button can help to scan large pages
- Use **Bookmarks** to record good sites
- You can search MEDLINE on the Internet at various sites, including PubMed: **http://www3.ncbi.nlm.nih.gov/PubMed/**

TCP/IP (Transmission Control Protocol / Internet Protocol): the lingua franca, a common language of protocols which allows different computers to exchange information.

- It is a loose association of networks of computers which has generated a massive publishing and communications arena.

- Every computer on the Internet (host) has its own unique IP address which defines where it is and enables other computers to send and forward messages to it. There is no central server for the Internet, so it is both robust (nearly impossible to destroy) and chaotic (nearly impossible to control).

- Typically, you will use your computer to log in to a host which has an Internet connection and which has an account for your use. If you are lucky, your machine will be a host in itself, which means others can log in to your machine and use it (for example, see Telnet).

- You will use the Internet from a particular domain (locality) which will have local management of services.

- The set of five services which are supported by the Internet protocols are:

E-mail (SMTP)	Text messages sent to a person: **user@host.domain**	User decides when to read, one to many with mailing lists, e.g. mailbase.	Not 100% reliable; Internet e-mail not universal in NHS; addresses can be obscure.
USENET News Groups (NNTP)	USENET servers contain textual discussion lists where users add their comments to a discussion.	Thousands of topics to choose from; can be a good source of advice.	Difficult to find relevant group; can be a source of abuse!
Telnet	Allows you to connect to a host computer across the Internet and use it as if you were sitting in front of it.	Allows you to use the resources of the host computer.	Usually just text-based commands, i.e. no Windows; you need an account with the host to be able to do this.
File transfer protocol (FTP)	You can log on to a host, browse its directories and exchange files efficiently (including programs).	You don't need authorization (anonymous FTP means you type 'Guest' as a login name and your e-mail address as password).	Can be very difficult to browse effectively (you have to know where to look and download to see what you are getting).
WWW (http)	Use a browser program to read multimedia documents (and programs) stored on any Internet host running the http program.	Instant publishing. Login, addressing and downloading with one click of the mouse. Can be searched and marked.	Imagine the Bodleian with all the books shuffled and dumped on the floor.

Usually, different services will be managed locally by a specific host (a server) which may or may not be the same machine.

Reference
Krol E (1994) The Whole Internet: users' guide and catalogue. O'Reilly.

PART A Presentations (comfortably 3 per hour)

1 In groups of 10 or less, participants will present their critical appraisals they have carried out on clinical topics of their choice.

2 Reports will state the 3-part clinical question, summarise the search in 1 sentence, critically appraise the best article found, and discuss how the appraisal was integrated with clinical expertise and applied on that (or a similar, subsequent) patient.

3 A total of 15 minutes will be allotted for each presentation: 10 minutes for presentation and 5 minutes for group discussion.

EBM SESSION

6

Presentations & searching the Cochrane Library

PART B Searching for evidence in the Cochrane Library

We will show you how to search the Cochrane Library (an electronic database of about 100 systematic reviews by the Cochrane Collaboration, abstracts of about 1,000 other systematic reviews from the world literature, citations for almost 180,000 randomised trials, and lots of information about the Cochrane Collaboration).

The Cochrane Library can be ordered from Update Software Ltd, Summertown Pavillion, Middle Way, Summertown, Oxford OX2 7LG; Tel: 01865 513902; Fax: 01865 516918; or via the Website at the Centre for Evidence-based Medicine: http://cebm.jr2.ox.ac.uk/

PART A — Presentations

The other half of the participants will present their patients, questions, critically appraised topics, and clinical conclusions.

PART B — Feedback and celebration

The final portion of the session (and course!) can be spent evaluating the course. The first of the attached forms (**Evaluation of 'practising EBM'**) permits written feedback about this course, and a discussion will be held on the general issues within it.

The second form (**'Am I practising EBM?'**) is a checklist that you may want to apply to your own performance in order to determine whether you are beginning to apply the self-directed, problem-based learning and EBM skills in your own practice and in your clinical teaching.

Special attention will be given to discussing and deciding what to do with what has been learned, and how to continue to improve and use this set of clinical, EBM and self-directed learning skills.

EVALUATION OF 'PRACTISING EBM'

Please rate the items using the following scale from 1 to 5 where:

1 – awful   3 – adequate   5 – excellent

1 *How well were your objectives met in this course?*

   a Learning how to ask answerable clinical questions related to pts
      you care for on the clinical service

      | | 1 | 2 | 3 | 4 | 5 |

   b Learning how to search for the best evidence

      | | 1 | 2 | 3 | 4 | 5 |

   c Learning how to critically appraise the medical literature

      | | 1 | 2 | 3 | 4 | 5 |

   d Learning how to integrate this literature with your clinical
      expertise and to apply the results in your clinical practice

      | | 1 | 2 | 3 | 4 | 5 |

   e Learning how to evaluate your performance

      | | 1 | 2 | 3 | 4 | 5 |

2 *Therapy Session*

	1	2	3	4	5
a Relevance of the session	1	2	3	4	5
b Appropriateness of the article	1	2	3	4	5
c Organisation of the session	1	2	3	4	5
d Teaching during the session	1	2	3	4	5

3 *Diagnosis Session*

	1	2	3	4	5
a Relevance of the session	1	2	3	4	5
b Appropriateness of the article	1	2	3	4	5
c Organisation of the session	1	2	3	4	5
d Teaching during the session	1	2	3	4	5

3 *Prognosis Session*

	1	2	3	4	5
a Relevance of the session	1	2	3	4	5
b Appropriateness of the article	1	2	3	4	5
c Organisation of the session	1	2	3	4	5
d Teaching during the session	1	2	3	4	5

4 *Systematic Review Session*

	1	2	3	4	5
a Relevance of the session	1	2	3	4	5
b Appropriateness of the article	1	2	3	4	5
c Organisation of the session	1	2	3	4	5
d Teaching during the session	1	2	3	4	5

5 *Harm Session*

    a Relevance of the session   1   2   3   4   5

    b Appropriateness of the article 1   2   3   4   5

    c Organisation of the session   1   2   3   4   5

    d Teaching during the session   1   2   3   4   5

6 *Final Presentation Sessions*

    a Relevance of the presentations 1   2   3   4   5

    b Quality of the presentations   1   2   3   4   5

    c Quality of the discussions   1   2   3   4   5

    d Organisation of the session   1   2   3   4   5

7 *How well do you think this course will help you prepare for your Membership Exams ?*

                               1   2   3   4   5

8 *Overall rating of the course*

                               1   2   3   4   5

9 *What was the best thing about this course
(that should be preserved and expanded in future courses)?*

10 *What was the worst thing about this course
(that should be removed from future courses of this sort)?*

11 *Other comments and suggestions:*

Many thanks

AM I PRACTISING EBM?

A self-evaluation in asking answerable questions.

a Are you asking any questions at all?

b Are you:

  • using the guides to ask 3-part questions?

  • using educational prescriptions

  • asking your colleagues: 'What's your evidence for that?'

c Is your success rate of asking answerable questions rising?

d How do your questions compare with those of respected colleagues?

A self-evaluation in finding the best external evidence.

a Are you searching at all?

b Do you know the best sources of current evidence for your clinical discipline?

c Have you achieved immediate access to searching hardware, software and the best evidence for your clinical discipline?

d Are you finding useful external evidence from a widening array of sources?

e Are you becoming more efficient in your searching?

f Are you using MeSH headings, thesaurus, limiters, and intelligent free text when searching MEDLINE?

g How do your searches compare with those of research librarians or other respected colleagues who have a passion for providing best current patient care?

A self-evaluation in critically appraising the evidence for its validity and potential usefulness.

a Are you critically appraising external evidence at all?

b Are the critical appraisal guides becoming easier to apply?

c Are you becoming more accurate and efficient in applying some of the critical appraisal measures (such as likelihood ratios, NNTs and the like)?

d Are you creating any CATs?

e Are you using the CATMaker?

f Have you shared any of the CATs you've made with your colleagues or other learners?

A self-evaluation in integrating the critical appraisal with your clinical expertise and applying the result in your clinical practice.

a Are you integrating your critical appraisals into your practice at all?

b Are you becoming more accurate and efficient in adjusting some of the critical appraisal measures to fit your individual patients (pre-test probabilities, NNT/f, etc.)?

c Can you explain (and resolve) disagreements about management decisions in terms of this integration?

d Have you conducted any clinical decision analyses?

e Have you carried out any audits of your diagnostic, therapeutic, or other EBM performance?

A self-evaluation in teaching EBM.

a   When did you last issue an educational prescription?

b   Are you helping your trainees learn how to ask answerable (3-part) questions?

c   Are you teaching and modelling searching skills (or making sure that your trainees learn them)?

d   Are you teaching and modelling critical appraisal skills?

e   Are you teaching and modelling the generation of CATs?

f   Are you teaching and modelling the integration of best evidence with individual clinical expertise?

g   Are you developing new ways of evaluating the effectiveness of your teaching?[1]

h   Are you developing new EBM educational materials?[2]

A self-evaluation of your own continuing professional development.

a   Are you a member of an EBM-style journal club?

b   Have you participated in or tutored at one of the workshops on how to practice or teach EBM?

c   Have you joined the evidence-based-health e-mail discussion group?

d   Have you established links with other practitioners or teachers of EBM?

[1] If so, please share them with the developers of this course!

[2] If so, please add them to the bank of EBM educational resources that the Oxford Centre for Evidence-based Medicine shares with other educators around the world.

Glossary of terms you are likely to encounter in your clinical reading

This glossary is intended to provide guidance as to the meanings of terms you will come across frequently in clinical articles, especially when they appear in EBM journals.

Absolute risk reduction (ARR) – see ***Treatment effects***

Case-control study – a study which involves identifying patients who have the outcome of interest (cases) and control patients without the same outcome, and looking back to see if they had the exposure of interest (*see also **Review of study designs***).

Case-series – a report on a series of patients with an outcome of interest. No control group is involved.

Clinical practice guideline – is a systematically developed statement designed to assist practitioner and patient decisions about appropriate health care for specific clinical circumstances.

Cohort study – involves identification of two groups (cohorts) of patients, one which did receive the exposure of interest, and one which did not, and following these cohorts forward for the outcome of interest (*see also **Review of study designs***).

Confidence interval (CI) – the range within which we would expect the true value of a statistical measure to lie. The CI is usually accompanied by a percentage value which shows the level of confidence that the true value lies within this range. For example, for an NNT of 10 with a 95% CI of 5 to 15, we would have 95% confidence that the true NNT value was between 5 and 15.

Control event rate (CER) – see ***Treatment effects***.

Cost-benefit analysis – assesses whether the cost of an intervention is worth the benefit by measuring both in the same units; monetary units are usually used.

Cost-effectiveness analysis – measures the net cost of providing a service as well as the outcomes obtained. Outcomes are reported in a single unit of measurement

Cost-utility analysis – converts effects into personal preferences (or utilities) and describes how much it costs for some additional quality gain (e.g. cost per additional quality-adjusted life-year, or QALY).

Crossover study design – the administration of two or more experimental therapies one after the other in a specified or random order to the same group of patients (*see also **Review of study designs***).

Cross-sectional study – the observation of a defined population at a single point in time or time interval. Exposure and outcome are determined simultaneously (*see also **Review of study designs***).

Decision analysis – is the application of explicit, quantitative methods that quantify prognoses, treatment effects, and patient values in order to analyse a decision under conditions of uncertainty.

Ecological survey – a survey based on aggregated data for some population as it exists at some point or points in time; to investigate the relationship of an exposure to a known or presumed risk factor for a specified outcome.

Event rate – the proportion of patients in a group in whom the event is observed. Thus, if out of 100 patients, the event is observed in 27, the event rate is 0.27. Control event rate (CER) and experimental event rate (EER) are used to refer to this in control and experimental groups of patients respectively. The patient expected event rate (PEER) refers to the rate of events we'd expect in a patient who received no treatment or conventional treatment – see **Treatment Effects**.

Evidence-based health care – extends the application of the principles of evidence-based medicine (see below) to all professions associated with health care, including purchasing and management.

Evidence-based medicine – the conscientious, explicit and judicious use of current best evidence in making decisions about the care of individual patients. The practice of evidence-based medicine means integrating individual clinical expertise with the best available external clinical evidence from systematic research. See also Sackett et al. (1996) EBM: What it is and what it isn't. BMJ **312:** 71–2.

Experimental event rate (EER) – see **Treatment effects**.

Likelihood ratio (LR) – the likelihood that a given test result would be expected in a patient with the target disorder compared to the likelihood that that same result would be expected in a patient without the target disorder.

Calculation of sensitivity/specificity/LR:

	DISEASE POSITIVE	DISEASE NEGATIVE
TEST POSITIVE	a	b
TEST NEGATIVE	c	d

Sensitivity = a/(a+c)

$$LR+ = \frac{sensitivity}{1-specificity} = \frac{a/(a+c)}{b/(b+d)}$$

Specificity = d/(b+d)

$$LR- = \frac{(1-sensitivity)}{specificity} = \frac{c/(a+c)}{d/(b+d)}$$

Positive predictive value = a/(a+b)   Negative predictive value = d/(c+d)

Meta-analysis – is an overview that uses quantitative methods to summarise the results.

N-of-1 trials – in such trials, the patient undergoes pairs of treatment periods organised so that one period involves the use of the experimental treatment and one period involves the use of an alternate or placebo therapy. The patients and physician are blinded, if possible, and outcomes are monitored. Treatment periods are replicated until the clinician and patient are convinced that the treatments are definitely different or definitely not different.

Negative predictive value – proportion of people with a negative test who are free of the target disorder (*see also* **Likelihood ratio**).

Number needed to treat (NNT) – is the inverse of the absolute risk reduction and is the number of patients that need to be treated to prevent one bad outcome – *see* **Treatment effects**.

Odds – a ratio of non-events to events. If the event rate for a disease is 0.1 (10%), its non-event rate is 0.9 and therefore its odds are 9:1. Note that this is not the same expression as the inverse of event rate.

Odds ratio (OR) – is the odds of having the target disorder in the experimental group relative to the odds in favour of having the target disorder in the control group (in prospective case-control studies, overviews) or the odds in favour of being exposed in subjects with the target disorder divided by the odds in favour of being exposed in control subjects (without the target disorder).

Calculations of OR/RR for use of trimethoprim-sulfamethoxazole prophylaxis in cirrhosis:

	Adverse event occurs (infectious complication)	Adverse event does not occur (no infectious complication)	Totals
Exposed to treatment (experimental)	1	29	30
	a	b	a+b
Not exposed to treatment (control)	c	d	c+d
	9	21	30
Totals	a+c	b+d	a+b+c+d
	10	50	60

CER = c/(c+d) = 0.30
EER= a/(a+b) = 0.033
Control Event Odds = c/d = 0.43
Experimental Event Odds = a/b = 0.034
Relative Risk = EER/CER = 0.11
Relative Odds = Odds Ratio = (a/b)/(c/d) = ad/bc = 0.08

Patient expected event rate – *see **Treatment effects***.

Overview – is a systematic review and summary of the medical literature (*see **meta analysis***).

Positive predictive value – proportion of people with a positive test who have the target disorder (*see also **Likelihood ratio***).

Randomised controlled clinical trial (RCT) – a group of patients is randomised into an experimental group and a control group. These groups are followed up for the variables / outcomes of interest (*see also **Review of study designs***).

Relative risk reduction (RRR) – *see **Treatment effects***.

Risk ratio (RR) – is the ratio of risk in the treated group (EER) to the risk in the control group (CER) – used in randomised trials and cohort studies:

$$RR = EER/CER$$

Sensitivity – proportion of people with the target disorder who have a positive test. It is used to assist in assessing and selecting a diagnostic test/sign/symptom (*see also **Likelihood ratio***).

SnNout – when a sign/test/symptom has a high **S**ensitivity, a **N**egative result rules **out** the diagnosis, e.g. the sensitivity of a history of ankle swelling for diagnosing ascites is 93%, therefore if a person does not have a history of ankle swelling, it is highly unlikely that the person has ascites.

Specificity – proportion of people without the target disorder who have a negative test. It is used to assist in assessing and selecting a diagnostic test/sign/symptom (*see also **Likelihood ratio***).

SpPin – when a sign/test/symptom has a high **S**pecificity, a **P**ositive result rules **in** the diagnosis, e.g. the specificity of a fluid wave for diagnosing ascites is 92%, therefore if a person does have a fluid wave, it rules in the diagnosis of ascites.

Systematic review – *see **Overview***.

Treatment effects

The E-B journals have achieved consensus on some terms they use to describe both the good and the bad effects of therapy. They will join the terms already in current use (RRR, ARR, NNT), and both sets are described here and summarised in the Glossary that appears inside the back cover of *Evidence-based Medicine*. We will bring them to life with a synthesis of three randomised trials in diabetes which individually showed that several years of intensive insulin therapy reduced the proportion of patients with worsening retinopathy to 13% from 38%, raised the proportion of patients with satisfactory haemoglobin A1c levels to 60% from about 30%, and increased the proportion of patients with at least one episode of symptomatic hypoglycaemia to 47% from 23%. Note that in each case the first number constitutes the 'experimental event rate' or EER and the second number the 'control event rate' or CER. We will use the following terms and calculations to describe these effects of treatment:

When the experimental treatment reduces the probability of a bad outcome (worsening diabetic retinopathy).

RRR (Relative risk reduction): the proportional reduction in rates of bad outcomes between experimental and control participants in a trial, calculated as lEER-CERl/CER, and accompanied by a 95% confidence interval (CI). In the case of worsening diabetic retinopathy, lEER-CERl/CER = l13%-38%l/38% = 66%.

ARR (Absolute risk reduction): the absolute arithmetic difference in rates of bad outcomes between experimental and control participants in a trial, calculated as lEER-CERl, and accompanied by a 95% CI. In this case, lEER-CERl =l13%-38%l = 25%.

NNT (Number needed to treat): the number of patients who need to be treated to achieve one additional favourable outcome, calculated as 1/ARR and accompanied by a 95% CI. In this case, 1/ARR = 1/25% = 4.

Calculations for the occurrence of diabetic retinopathy in IDDMs:

Occurrence of diabetic neuropathy at 5 yr among insulin-dependent diabetics in the DCCT trial		Relative risk reduction (RRR)	Absolute risk reduction (ARR)	Number needed to treat (NNT)
Usual insulin regimen CER	Intensive insulin regimen EER	$\frac{\text{lEER–CERl}}{\text{CER}}$	lEER–CERl	1/ARR
13%	38%	$\frac{\text{l13\%-38\%l} = 66\%}{38\%}$	l13%-38%l =25%	1/25%= 4 pts, for 6 years, with intensive insulin Rx

When the experimental treatment increases the probability of a good outcome (satisfactory haemoglobin A1c levels).

RBI (Relative benefit increase): the proportional increase in rates of good outcomes between experimental and control patients in a trial, calculated as lEER-CERl/CER, and accompanied by a 95% confidence interval (CI). In the case of satisfactory haemoglobin A1c levels, lEER-CERl/CER =l60%-30%l/30% = 100%.

ABI (Absolute benefit increase): the absolute arithmetic difference in rates of good outcomes between experimental and control patients in a trial, calculated as lEER-CERl, and accompanied by a 95% CI. In the case of satisfactory haemoglobin A1c levels, lEER-CERl = l60%–30%l =30%.

NNT (Number needed to treat): the number of patients who need to be treated to achieve one additional good outcome, calculated as 1/ARR and accompanied by a 95% CI. In this case, 1/ARR = 1/30% = 3.

When the experimental treatment increases the probability of a bad outcome (episodes of hypoglycaemia).

RRI (Relative risk increase): the proportional increase in rates of bad outcomes between experimental and control patients in a trial, calculated as IEER-CERI/CER, and accompanied by a 95% CI. In the case of hypoglycaemic episodes, IEER-CERI/CER = I57%-23%I/57% = 34%/57% = 60%. (RRI is also used in assessing the impact of 'risk factors' for disease.)

ARI (Absolute risk increase): the absolute arithmetic difference in rates of bad outcomes between experimental and control patients in a trial, calculated as IEER-CERI, and accompanied by a 95% CI. In the case of hypoglycaemic episodes, IEER-CERI = I57%-23%I = 34%. (ARI is also used in assessing the impact of 'risk factors' for disease.)

NNH (Number needed to harm): the number of patients who, if they received the experimental treatment, would lead to one additional patient being harmed, compared with patients who received the control treatment, calculated as 1/ARR and accompanied by a 95% CI. In this case, 1/ARR = 1/34% = 3.

		Adverse Outcome		Totals
		Present (Case)	**Absent (Control)**	
Exposed to the Treatment	Yes (Cohort)	a	b	a+b
	No (Cohort)	c	d	c+d
	Totals	a+c	b+d	a+b+c+d

In a randomised trial or cohort study:
Relative risk = RR = [a/(a+b)]/[c/(c+d)]

In a case-control study:
Odds ratio (or Relative odds) = OR = ad/bc

Randomized controlled trial: start with a+b+c+d and randomise to (a+b) and (c+d)

Advantages

1 Assignment to treatment can be kept concealed.
2 Confounders equally distributed.
3 Blinding more likely.
4 Randomisation facilitates statistical analysis.

Disadvantages

1 Expensive – time and money.
2 Volunteer bias.
3 Ethically problematic at times.

Crossover design

Advantages

1 Subjects serve as own controls and error variance is reduced thus reducing sample size needed.
2 All subjects receive treatment (at least some of the time).
3 Statistical tests assuming randomisation can be used.
4 Blinding can be maintained.

Disadvantages

1 All subjects receive placebo or alternative treatment at some point.
2 Washout period lengthy or unknown.
3 Cannot be used for treatments with permanent effects.

Cohort study: selects (a+b) and (c+d)

Advantages
1 Ethically safe.
2 Subjects can be matched.
3 Can establish timing and direction of events.
4 Eligibility criteria and outcome assessments can be standardised.
5 Administratively easier and cheaper than RCT.

Disadvantages
1 Controls may be difficult to identify.
2 Exposure may be linked to a hidden confounder.
3 Blinding difficult.
4 Still expensive.
5 Randomisation not present.
6 For rare disease, large sample sizes or long follow-up necessary.

Cross-sectional (analytic) survey: selecting a+b+c+d

Advantages
1 Cheap and simple.
2 Safe ethically.

Disadvantages
1 Establishes association at most, not causality.
2 Recall bias susceptibility.
3 Confounders may be unequally distributed.
4 Neyman bias.
5 Group sizes may be unequal.

Case-control study: selecting (a+c) and (b+d)

Advantages
1 Quick and cheap.
2 Only feasible method for very rare disorders or those with long lag between exposure and outcome
3 Fewer subjects needed than cross-sectional studies

Disadvantages
1 Reliance on recall or records to determine exposure status.
2 Confounders.
3 Selection of control groups difficult.
4 Potential bias – recall, selection.

Evidence-based Medicine

Section 3a1

Is this evidence about a diagnostic test valid?

Having found a possibly useful article about a diagnostic test, how can you quickly critically appraise it for its proximity to the truth? This can be done by asking some simple questions; often you'll find their answers in the article's abstract. Table 3a1.1 lists these questions for individual reports, but you can also apply them to the interpretation of a systematic review (overview) of several different studies of the same diagnostic test for the same target disorder.*

The first guide is: 'Was there an independent, blind comparison with a reference ("gold") standard of diagnosis?' This is quite a mouthful, but it simply means that two criteria should have been met. The patients in the study should have undergone *both* the diagnostic test in question (say, an item of the history or physical examination, a blood test, etc.) *and* the reference (or 'gold') standard (an autopsy or biopsy or other confirmatory 'proof' that they do or don't have the target disorder); and the results of one shouldn't be known to those who are applying and interpreting the other (for example, the pathologist interpreting the biopsy that comprises the reference standard for the target disorder should be 'blind' to the result of the blood test that comprises the diagnostic test under study). In this way, investigators avoid the conscious and unconscious bias that otherwise might cause the reference standard to be 'overinterpreted' when the diagnostic test is positive and 'underinterpreted' when it is negative. Sometimes investigators have a difficult time coming up with clearcut

* As we'll stress throughout this book, systematic reviews will give you the most valid and useful external evidence on just about any clinical question you can pose. They are still pretty rare for diagnostic tests and for this reason we'll describe them in their usual, therapeutic habitat, in Section 3a3. When using Table 3a3.2 to consider diagnostic tests, simply substitute 'diagnostic test' for 'treatment' as you read.

Table 3a1.1 Are the results of this diagnostic study valid?

1. Was there an independent, blind comparison with a reference ('gold') standard of diagnosis?
2. Was the diagnostic test evaluated in an appropriate spectrum of patients (like those in whom it would be used in practice)?
3. Was the reference standard applied regardless of the diagnostic test result?

reference standards (e.g. for psychiatric disorders) and you'll want to give careful consideration to their arguments justifying the selection of their reference standard.

One way or another, the report will wind up calling some results 'normal' and others 'abnormal' and we'll show you how to interpret these in Section 3b1. For now, you might simply want to recognize that there are six definitions of 'normal' in common use (we've listed them in Table 3a1.2). We will make use of definition 5 ('diagnostic' normal) and believe that half of the definitions are not useful. The first two (the Gaussian and percentile definitions) are derived from the study test results alone, with no reference standard, and simply define the 'normal range' for the diagnostic test result on the basis of statistical properties (standard deviations or percentiles). Thus they are properties of the test in isolation from any objective reality. These don't make any sense to us, for they imply that all 'abnormalities' occur at the same frequency. They both suggest that if we can perform enough diagnostic tests on a patient we are bound to find something 'abnormal' and lead to all sorts of inappropriate further testing. The third definition of 'normal' (culturally desirable) represents a cultural value judgment. It is seen in fashion advertisements and at the fringes of the 'lifestyle' movement where medicine becomes confused with morality. The fourth (risk factor) definition has the drawback that it 'labels' or stigmatizes some patients and is clinically useful only if we can do something positive to lower their risk. The fifth (diagnostic) definition is the one that we will focus on here and we will show you how to generate and interpret diagnostic normality in Section 3b1. The final (therapeutic) definition is in part an outgrowth of the

Table 3a1.2 Six definitions of normal

1. Gaussian: the mean +/- 2 standard deviations. Assumes a normal distribution and means that all 'abnormalities' have the same frequency.
2. Percentile: within the range, say, of 5–95%. Has the same basic defect as the Gaussian definition.
3. Culturally desirable: preferred by society. Confuses the role of medicine.
4. Risk factor: carrying no additional risk of disease. Labels the outliers, who may not be helped.
5. Diagnostic: range of results beyond which target disorders become highly probable – the focus of this discussion.
6. Therapeutic: range of results beyond which treatment does more good than harm. Means you have to keep up with advances in therapy!

fourth (risk factor) definition and has the great clinical advantage that it changes with our knowledge of efficacy. Thus, the definition of normal blood pressure has changed radically over the past few decades as we have learned that treatment of progressively lower blood pressure levels does more good than harm.

Returning to the second question in Table 3a1.1, you will want the diagnostic test to have been evaluated in an appropriate spectrum of patients, similar to the practice population in which the test might be used. Among patients with late or severe disease, when the diagnosis is obvious, often you won't need any diagnostic test, so studies that confine themselves to florid cases are not very informative. The article will be informative if the diagnostic test was applied to patients with mild as well as severe and early as well as late cases of the target disorder and among both treated and untreated individuals. In addition, you would want the diagnostic test to have been applied to patients with different disorders that are commonly confused with the target disorder of interest.

Finally, was the reference standard applied regardless of the diagnostic test result? When patients have a negative diagnostic test result, investigators are tempted to forego applying the reference standard and when the latter is invasive or risky (e.g. angiography) it may be considered inappropriate

Section 3a2

Is this evidence about prognosis valid?

Clinicians consider questions about prognosis all the time. Sometimes the questions are posed by patients and are quite direct (How long have I got?). At other times the questions are posed by clinicians and are indirect, as when deciding *whether* to treat at all (e.g. an elderly man with chronic lymphocyte leukemia who feels well – would his prognosis be importantly altered if he were left alone until he becomes symptomatic?) or deciding *whether* to screen (e.g. for abdominal aortic aneurysms – what is the fate of the undetected 4 cm aneurysm?). These questions share two elements: a qualitative aspect (Which outcomes could happen?) and a temporal aspect (Over what time period?). In Chapter 1 we showed you how to recognize such questions as being about prognosis and in Chapter 2 we addressed how to find good information about prognosis. In this part of Chapter 3 we'll present a framework for appraising the validity and importance of evidence about prognosis, for use when you tackle situations like the ones above (see Table 3a2.1). We'll consider them in sequence.

The four guides that will help you decide whether some evidence about prognosis is valid are listed in Table 3a2.1. First of all, was a defined, representative sample of patients assembled at a common (usually early) point in the course of their disease? Ideally, the prognosis study you find would include the entire population of patients who ever lived who developed the disease, studied from the instant of its onset. Since this is impossible, you'll want to look at how far from ideal will still tell you what you need to know and you'll do that by finding the methods section (if there isn't one, maybe you're wasting your time on this report!) and reading how the study patients were assembled. You'd want their illness to be defined well enough for you to be clear about it and you'd want the entire spectrum of severity that would occur at that common point to be represented.

Table 3a2.1 Is this evidence about prognosis valid?

1. Was a defined, representative sample of patients assembled at a common (usually early) point in the course of their disease?
2. Was patient follow-up sufficiently long and complete?
3. Were objective outcome criteria applied in a 'blind' fashion?
4. If subgroups with different prognoses are identified:
   - Was there adjustment for important prognostic factors?
   - Was there validation in an independent group of 'test-set' patients?

But when should the 'clock start'? That is, from what point in the disease should patients be followed? If investigators begin tracking outcomes only *after* several patients have already finished their course with the disease, then the outcomes for these patients would never be counted. Some would have recovered quickly, whilst others might have died quickly. So, to avoid missing outcomes by 'starting the clock' too late, you should look to see that study patients were included at a uniformly early time in the disease, ideally when it first becomes clinically manifest, the so-called 'inception cohort'. An exception might be if you wanted to learn about the prognosis of a late stage in the disease (e.g. for clinically manifest coronary heart disease); in this case you'd look for a representative and well-defined sample of patients who were all at at a similarly advanced stage (e.g. when they had their first clinical coronary event, not when they first developed elevated coronary risk factors).

Second, was patient follow-up sufficiently long and complete? Ideally, every patient in the inception cohort would be followed over time until they fully recover or one of the disease outcomes occurs. If with short follow-up few study patients have any of the outcomes of interest, you won't have enough to go on when advising your patients. Of course, if after decades of follow-up few adverse events have occurred, this good prognostic result is very useful in reassuring your patient about the future. If you think that the follow-up is too short to have developed a valid picture of the extent of the outcome of your interest, you'd better look for other evidence.

to do so. For this reason, many investigators now employ a reference standard for a patient *not* having the target disorder in which they *don't* suffer any adverse health outcome during a long follow-up on no definitive treatment (for example, convincing evidence that a patient with clinically suspected deep vein thrombosis did *not* have this disorder would be a prolonged follow-up on no antithrombotic therapy and suffering no ill effects).

If the report you're reading fails one or more of these three tests you'll need to consider whether it has a fatal flaw that renders its conclusions invalid; if so, it's back to more searching (either now or later; if you haven't enough time, perhaps you can interest a colleague or trainee in taking this on). If the report passes this initial scrutiny and you decide that you can believe its results, but you haven't already carried out the second critical appraisal step of deciding whether these results are impressive, then you can proceed to Section 3b1 on page 118.

Further reading

Jaeschke R, Guyatt G H, Sackett D L for the Evidence-Based Medicine Working Group. Users' guides to the medical literature. VI. How to use an article about a diagnostic test. A: Are the results of the study valid? JAMA 1994; 271: 389–91.

Evidence-based Medicine

If follow-up was long enough, you still have to worry about patients who entered the study but got lost along the way. Patients are almost always lost to follow-up and their outcomes will be excluded from the study's conclusions about prognosis. Some losses to follow-up are both unavoidable and unrelated to prognosis (e.g. moving away to a better job) and these aren't a cause for worry. But other losses might be because patients die or are too ill to continue follow-up (or lose their independence and move in with family) and the failure to document and report their outcomes will threaten the validity of the report. Short of finding a report that kept track of every patient, how can you judge whether follow-up is 'sufficiently complete'? There is no single answer for all studies, but we offer two suggestions to help you make this judgment. The first is a simple '5 and 20' rule of thumb: fewer than 5% loss probably leads to little bias, greater than 20% loss seriously threatens validity and in-between amounts cause intermediate amounts of trouble. While this may be easy to remember, it may oversimplify for clinical situations in which the outcomes are infrequent.

The second approach uses a 'worst-case' scenario. Imagine a study of prognosis wherein 100 patients enter the study, four die and 16 are lost to follow-up. A 'crude' survival rate would count the four deaths among the 84 with total follow-up, for a death rate of 4.8%, and then report a survival rate of $100\% - 4.8\% = 95.2\%$. But what of the lost 16? Some or all of them might have died too. The latter, 'worst-case' scenario would mean a case-fatality rate of (four known + 16 lost) or 20 out of (84 followed up + 16 lost) or 20/100, that is 20% (four times the observed rate!); note that in order to determine the 'worst-case' scenario you've added the lost patients to both the numerator and denominator of the outcome rate. On the other hand, in the 'best-case' scenario none of the lost 16 would have died, yielding a case-fatality rate of 4 out of (84 + 16) or 4/100, that is 4%; note that in determining the 'best-case' scenario you add the missing cases to just the denominator. While this 'best case' of 4% may not differ much from the observed 4.8%, the 'worst case' of 20% does differ meaningfully and you'd probably judge that this study's follow-up

was not sufficiently complete. By seeing what effect the losses might have on the result you can decide whether a 'worst-case' scenario would change your conclusion about prognosis. If this simple form of 'sensitivity analysis' suggests that losses wouldn't change the result much, then you can judge the follow-up as sufficiently complete.

You can use these first two guides to screen articles about prognosis to find the few worth more of your limited time. If you've answered 'no' to both of the above questions, you can be pretty sure the study will not provide estimates of prognosis that are close to the truth and you ought to start searching for better evidence. If, on the other hand, you've answered 'yes' to both of the above questions, you can be reasonably confident that the study will provide accurate information about prognosis. To be even more sure of this, you should ask the remaining two validity questions in Table 3a2.1.

Were objective outcome criteria applied in a 'blind' fashion? Diseases can affect patients in many important ways; some are easy to spot and some are more subtle. In general, outcomes at both extremes, death or full recovery, are relatively easy to detect and be sure of. In between these extremes are a wide range of outcomes that can be more difficult to detect or confirm and where investigators will have to use judgment in deciding how to count them up. Examples include the degree of disease activity/quiescence, the readiness for return to work and the intensity of residual pain. To minimize the effects of bias, investigators can establish specific criteria that define each possible outcome of the disease and then use these criteria during patient follow-up. You can usually find such outcome criteria in the text, tables, appendices or references in the study. You should satisfy yourself that they are sufficiently objective for confirming the outcomes you're interested in. The occurrence of death is about as objective as you can get, but judging the underlying cause of death is very prone to error (especially when it's based on death certificates) and can be biased unless objective criteria are applied to high-quality clinical evidence.

But even with objective criteria, some bias might creep in if the investigators judging the outcomes also know the

patients' characteristics. To minimize this bias, the authors of the report should have taken precautions so that the investigators making judgments about clinical outcomes were 'blind' to these patients' clinical characteristics and prognostic factors. The more subjective the outcome, the more important such blinding becomes. You should satisfy yourself that blinding was used if it would have been important for the outcomes of interest to you.

The final pair of guides have to do with reports that claim that one subgroup of patients has a different prognosis from others. Such reports are common and for good clinical reason. Often you will want to know whether subgroups of patients have different prognoses (e.g. among patients with non-valvular atrial fibrillation, are those with enlarged left atria at higher risk for stroke than those with normal sized atria?). The first guide here suggests that you look to see whether there was adjustment for other important prognostic factors. That is, reports that address this sort of question should have made sure that these subgroup predictions aren't being distorted by the unequal occurrence of another, powerful prognostic factor (such as would occur if patients with large atria were also more likely to have had prior embolic stroke than patients with normal atria). There are both simple (e.g. stratified analyses displaying the prognoses of patients with large atria separately for those with and without prior embolic stroke) and fancy (e.g. multiple regression analyses that could take into account not only prior embolic stroke but also hypertension, left ventricular function and the like) ways of adjusting for these other important prognostic factors and you should reassure yourself that one or the other has been applied before you tentatively accept the conclusion about a different prognosis for the subgroup of interest.

We say tentatively because there is one final guide to deciding whether a claim that a subgroup has a different prognosis should be accepted as valid. This is the fact that the statistics of determining subgroup prognoses are all about prediction, not explanation. They are indifferent to whether the prognostic factor is physiologically logical (in our running example, whether the left atrial size) or biologically nonsensical (whether the

The main questions to answer:
1. Was the assignment of patients to treatments randomized? and was the randomization list concealed?
2. Were all patients who entered the trial accounted for at its conclusion? and were they analyzed in the groups to which they were randomized?

And some finer points to address:
1. Were patients and clinicians kept 'blind' to which treatment was being received?
2. Aside from the experimental treatment, were the groups treated equally?
3. Were the groups similar at the start of the trial?

---

patient's navel is concave (an 'innie') or convex (an 'outie'). These prognostic factors can be demographic (such as age, gender, socioeconomic status), disease specific (such as extent of disease, degree of test abnormality) or comorbid (presence or absence of many other conditions). Keep in mind that these prognostic factors need not cause the outcome; they need only be associated with its development strongly enough to predict it.

For this reason, the first time a prognostic factor is identified, there is no guarantee it isn't the result of a random, non-causal 'quirk' in its distribution between patients with different prognoses; for that reason, the initial patient group in which it was identified is called a 'training set'. As you might imagine, if this initial study carried out a multivariate analysis looking for potential prognostic factors, they'd be very likely to find at least a few, just on the basis of chance (and most investigators would be imaginative enough to suggest logical explanations for them). Because of this risk of spurious, chance nomination of prognostic factors, you should seek its confirmation in a report of a second, independent group (called a 'test set') of patients. The best evidence for this is finding a statement (in the methods section) of a prestudy intention to examine this specific possible prognostic factor (based on its appearance in a training set). If that second, independent study also identifies the prognostic factor, you can feel much more confident that the evidence about it is valid.

If your evidence flunks these tests for validity, we're afraid it's back to searching, either now (if you still have time) or at a later session. If, on a happier note, you decide that the evidence you've found about a prognostic factor is valid and you haven't already decided whether it's also important, you can take that consideration up in Section 3b2 on page 129.

Further reading

Laupacis A, Wells G, Richardson W S, Tugwell P for the Evidence-Based Medicine Working Group. Users' guides to the medical literature. V. How to use an article about prognosis. JAMA 1994; 272: 234-7.

Section 3a3

Is this evidence about a treatment valid?

Having found some possibly useful evidence about therapy, you have to decide where to start in its critical appraisal. On the one hand, you could start here in Section 3a3, with an appraisal of its validity (arguing that if it's not valid, who cares whether it appears to show a big effect?). On the other, you could go right to determining its importance in Section 3b3 (arguing that if the evidence doesn't suggest a possibly useful clinical impact, who cares if it's valid?). Begin with either end and then pick up the other. This section will help you to quickly and critically appraise evidence about therapy for its closeness to the truth. This can be done by asking some simple questions and often you'll find their answers in an abstract that accompanies the evidence. Table 3a3.1 lists these questions for reports of individual therapeutic trials, but since these can best be interpreted in the context of all other trials on the same topic, Table 3a3.2 summarizes guides for assessing evidence that has combined the results of several trials into an overview or systematic review (when a systematic review uses special statistical methods for combining the results of several studies, we call it a meta-analysis). Alternatively, you may encounter (or have tracked down) an economic analysis, which is a more complex method that compares therapeutic alternatives from a broader perspective (including those of health managers or even society as a whole) and tries to offer or provide treatments in the way that best uses scarce resources such as hospital beds, drugs, operating time, clinicians and money. Questions pertinent to deciding whether you should believe an economic analysis appear in Table 3a3.3. Finally, and building on the earlier section on diagnosis, we'll give you a brief description of how to decide whether to believe evidence on the effects of therapy when it is formulated into a clinical decision analysis; rules for deciding whether to believe their results are described in Section 3a3.4.

When several randomized trials of the same treatment for the same condition have been carried out, we think you'll agree that an overview which systematically reviews and combines all of them would give you a better answer than a critical appraisal of just one of them. For that reason, we suggested back in Chapter 2 that you always start your search for useful clinical articles on just about any topic by looking for systematic reviews. However, because systematic reviews assess their component trials individually (and, as you can see in Table 3a3.2, you want to be sure that they've done that in a valid way) and since at this point in history you're much more likely to find individual trials than systematic reviews, we'll begin with the individual trial.

Is the evidence from this randomized trial valid?

We'll begin with two important questions:

1. Was the assignment of patients to treatments randomized and was the randomization schedule concealed?

When deciding whether the evidence from a randomized trial is valid, the most important question to ask (and frequently the quickest question to answer) is: Was the assignment of patients to treatments randomized? That is, was some method analogous to tossing a coin* used to assign patients to treatments (with the treatment you're interested in given if the coin landed 'heads' and a conventional, 'control' or placebo† treatment given if the coin landed 'tails')? The reason for insisting on random allocation to treatments is that this comes closer than any other research design to creating groups of patients at the start of the trial who are identical in their risk of the events you're hoping to prevent. It does this in two, related ways. First, the coin toss balances the groups for prognostic factors (such as disease severity or other predictors of especially good or bad prognosis) which, if they were unevenly distributed between treatment groups, could exaggerate, cancel or even counteract the effects of therapy.‡ If they exaggerated the apparent effects of an otherwise ineffectual treatment, the effects of their imbalance could lead to the false-positive conclusion that the treatment was useful when it was not. And if they cancelled or counteracted the effects of a really efficacious treatment, the effects of their imbalance could lead to the false-negative conclusion that a useful treatment was useless or even harmful. Random allocation balances the treatment groups for these and other prognostic factors, even if we don't yet understand the disorder well enough to know what they are!

The second, related benefit of random allocation is that, if it is concealed from the clinicians who are entering patients into the trial, they will be unaware of which treatment the next patient will receive and they can't either consciously or unconsciously distort the balance between the groups being compared. So you want to be sure that both of these standards are met. Usually it's easy to tell whether a study was

* In practice, this coin tossing is done by special computer programs, but the principle is exactly the same.
† A placebo is a treatment that is so similar in appearance, taste, etc. that the patient ('single-blind') or the clinician or both ('double-blind') are unable to distinguish it from the active treatment.
‡ 'Confounder' is a technical name for these sorts of patient characteristics that are extraneous to the question posed, could cause the clinical events we are trying to prevent with the treatment and might be unevenly distributed between the treatment groups. And although there are other ways of avoiding confounding (exclusion, stratified sampling, matching, stratified analysis, standardization and multivariate modelling), they all demand that you already know what the confounder is.

randomized, because it's something to be proud of and that term often appears in the title and almost always in the abstract. On the other hand, it's not often stated whether the randomization list was concealed, but if randomization occurred by telephone or by some system that was at a distance from where patients were being entered into the trial, you can be comfortable about this. If randomization wasn't concealed, this tends to lead to patients with more favourable prognoses being given the experimental treatment, exaggerating the apparent benefits of therapy and perhaps even leading to the false-positive conclusion that the treatment is efficacious when it is not.

If you find that the study was not randomized, we'd suggest that you stop reading it and go on to the next article. Only if you can't find any randomized trials should you come back and have another go at it. But if the only evidence you have about a treatment is from non-randomized studies, you are in a bind and have five options:

1. Check Chapter 2 again or get help in doing another literature search to see if you missed any randomized trials of the candidate therapy.
2. See whether the treatment effect is simply so huge that you can't imagine it could be a false-positive study (this usually happens only when the prognosis is uniformly awful and is a very rare situation). As a check, ask several colleagues whether they consider the candidate therapy so likely to be efficacious that they'd consider it unethical to randomize a patient like yours into a study of it that includes a no-treatment or placebo group.*
3. Conversely, if the non-randomized study concluded that the treatment was useless or harmful, then it is usually safe to accept that conclusion (since, as described above, false-negative conclusions from non-randomized studies are less likely than false-positive ones).
4. Consider whether an 'N-of-1' trial would make sense to you and your patient (they are described on page 173).

* This is the 'convincing non-experimental evidence' category used in the audits of clinical care reported on page 3 (the A-team study).

5. Try some other treatment or simply provide supportive care.

2. Were all patients who entered the trial accounted for at its conclusion and were they analysed in the groups to which they were randomized?

Having satisfied yourself that the trial really was randomized, you can then match the number of patients who entered the trial with the number accounted for at its conclusion. Ideally, these numbers will be identical, for lost patients could have had events that would change the conclusion. If, for example, patients on the experimental treatment dropped out and had adverse outcomes, their absence from the analysis would lead it to overestimate the efficacy of that treatment. What's an acceptable loss? To be sure of a trial's conclusion, its authors should be able to take all patients who were lost along the way, assign them the 'worst-case' outcomes (that is, assume that everyone lost from the group whose remaining members fared better had a bad outcome and assume that everyone lost from the group whose remaining members fared worse had a rosy outcome) and still be able to support their original conclusion. It would be unusual for a trial to withstand a worst-case analysis if it lost more than 20% of its patients and journals like *Evidence-Based Medicine* won't publish trials with <80% follow-up.

Because anything that happens after randomization can affect the chances that a patient in a trial has an event, it's important that all patients (even those who fail to take their medicine or accidentally or intentionally receive the wrong treatment) are analysed in the groups to which they were randomized. This is an essential prerequisite for valid evidence about the effects of therapy. For example, it has repeatedly been shown that patients who do and don't take their study medicine have very different outcomes, even when the study medicine they have been prescribed is a placebo! The correct form of analysis, in which patients are analysed in the groups to which they were assigned, is called an 'intention to treat' analysis.

There are three less important questions to ask when you are trying to decide whether a randomized trial has produced valid evidence:

1. Were patients and clinicians kept 'blind' to which treatment was being received?
2. Aside from the experimental treatment, were the groups treated equally?
3. Were the groups similar at the start of the trial?

If you decide that the study really was randomized, follow-up was virtually complete and patients were analyzed in the groups to which they'd been randomized, you can look for some other features that provide even greater assurance that you can believe its results. If, for example, it was a pharmacological trial in which patients received either a tablet containing the active drug or an identical-appearing (in size, shape, colour, taste, etc.) tablet of pharmacologically inert ingredients (a placebo), then it would be possible to keep both patients and clinicians blind* as to which treatment was received and neither the patient's reporting of symptoms nor the clinician's interpretation of them would be influenced by their hunches about whether the treatment was efficacious. Another advantage of the double-blind method is that it prevents patients and their clinicians from adding any additional treatments (or 'cointerventions') to just one of the groups. When patients and their clinicians can't be kept blind (as in surgical trials), often it is possible to have other, blinded clinicians come in and assess clinical records (purged of any mention of treatment) or make special outcome measurements. And finally, you can double-check to see whether randomization was effective by looking to see whether patients were similar at the start of the trial (most trials display this in the first table of their results).

Whether the results of an individual trial are important is considered in Section 3b3 on page 133.

---

* When patients don't know their treatment but their doctors do (as when the active drug causes a clearcut sign such as bradycardia), the trial is called 'single blind'. When both are blind, it is called 'double blind'.

Evidence-based Medicine

Is the evidence from this systematic review valid?

Having shown you how to decide whether to believe the results of a single trial, let's now turn to how you can decide whether to believe the results of an overview of several trials. The key questions you need to answer are in Table 3a3.2.

Table 3a3.2 Are the results of this systematic review valid?

1. Is it an overview of randomized trials of the treatment you're interested in?
2. Does it include a methods section that describes:
   a. finding and including all the relevant trials?
   b. assessing their individual validity?
3. Were the results consistent from study to study?

1. Is it a systematic review of randomized trials of the treatment you're interested in?

This first question asks whether you are sure that the treatment is the same as the one you're considering and immediately asking whether the overview is combining reports of studies carried out at the same, most powerful level of evidence that we've been discussing here, the randomized trial. Systematic reviews of non-randomized studies of therapy simply compound the problems of individually misleading trials and the same warnings apply. Moreover, some overviews combine randomized and non-randomized studies and unless the authors have provided separate information on the subset of randomized trials, you shouldn't trust them either.

2. Does it include a methods section that describes: (a) finding and including all the relevant trials; (b) assessing their individual validity?

You should see whether the overview report includes a methods section that describes how they found all the relevant trials and how they assessed their individual validity. Let's take these three elements one by one. First, because performing an overview is performing research (it involves posing a question, identifying a population and drawing a sample, making measurements, analyzing them and drawing

conclusions), it should be carried out and reported like research. If you don't find a methods section, be very wary of believing its results; maybe its only useful part will be its bibliography of individual trials for you to study as above. Second, if the overview has a methods section it should describe how its authors tracked down and included all the trials that were relevant to this treatment. This is no easy task. The standard bibliographic databases described in Chapter 2, good as they are, fail to correctly label up to half of the published trials and 'negative' trials (that conclude the treatment is not efficacious) are less likely to be submitted for publication, leading an overview of those that are published to overestimate the treatment's efficacy. Signs that the overviewers did a good job are positive when they report at least some hand searching of the most relevant journals (for miscoded trials) and especially when they report contacting the authors of published trials (who often will know about unpublished ones). Third, you should look for a statement of how they decided whether the individual trials in their overview were scientifically sound, using criteria like those in Table 3a3.1. Finally, because these last two steps of deciding which trials to include in the overview involve a lot of judgment calls, you should be especially reassured when you find that two or more investigators carried out these tasks independent of each other and achieved good agreement about their judgments.

3. Were the results consistent from study to study?

It stands to reason that we are more likely to believe an overview when the results of all the trials in it show a treatment effect going in the same direction. Although we shouldn't expect each of them to show exactly the same degree of efficacy (that is, we should be comfortable with a certain amount of quantitative difference in the trial results), we would be concerned if we found some trials in an overview confidently concluding a beneficial effect of the treatment and other trials confidently concluding no benefit or a harmful effect. Such a qualitative difference in the effects of treatment (which also goes by the name of heterogeneity), unless it can be explained to your satisfaction (such as by differences in patients or in doses or durations of treatment), should lead you to be very cautious about believing any overall conclusion about efficacy in all patients and you'd hope to see your caution expressed in the conclusions of the overview.

Whether the results of an overview are important is considered in Section 3b3 on page 133.

Section 3a4
Is this evidence about harm valid?

You must frequently make judgments on whether a treatment is harming or has harmed a patient. Many admissions to acute general hospitals are the result of adverse drug reactions and reactions to diagnostic and therapeutic maneuvers are judged to befall one-fifth to one-third of patients after they are admitted. On the other hand, even clinical pharmacologists disagree about whether a given patient has had an adverse drug reaction and the fact that an adverse reaction occurred *during* a treatment is insufficient evidence that it occurred *because* of that treatment.

Faced with a problem that is pandemic yet controvertible, clinicians must equip themselves to answer two related questions:

1. Does this drug (or operation or other treatment) cause that adverse effect in *some* patients? And, if so:
2. Did this drug (or operation or other treatment) cause that adverse effect in *this particular* patient?

This section will deal with the first question and the second question will be addressed in Section 4.4.

Because this assessment can be viewed as addressing a general question of *causation*, it benefits from what has been learned about asking and answering such questions in classical epidemiology. The four guides for deciding whether to believe the claim that a treatment harms some patients are summarized in Table 3a4.1, and we'll consider them in sequence.

1. Were there clearly defined groups of patients, similar in all important ways other than exposure to the treatment?

Because the 'threats to validity' are different for different sorts of studies, you'll have to spend just a little time sorting them out. Suppose you wanted to decide whether fenoterol (a beta-agonist used to treat asthma) sometimes harm

105

rarely) caused the death of its users. You could look for and find four different sorts of studies and all of them can be illustrated by reference to Table 3a4.2. First, you could look for a randomized trial in which asthma patients were assigned, by a system analogous to tossing a coin, to receive fenoterol (the top row in Table 3a4.2, whose total is **a+b**)

Table 3a4.1 Are the results of this harm study valid?

1. Were there clearly defined groups of patients, similar in all important ways other than exposure to the treatment?
2. Were treatment exposures and clinical outcomes measured in the same way in both groups?
3. Was the follow-up of study patients complete and long enough?
4. Do the results satisfy some 'diagnostic tests for causation'?
   • Is it clear that the exposure preceded the onset of the outcome?
   • Is there a dose-response gradient?
   • Is there positive evidence from a 'dechallenge–rechallenge' study?
   • Is the association consistent from study to study?
   • Does the association make biological sense?

	Adverse Outcome		Totals
	Present (Case)	Absent (Control)	
Exposed to the treatment — Yes (Cohort)	a	b	a+b
No (Cohort)	c	d	c+d
Totals	a+c	b+d	a+b+c+d

Table 3a4.2 Different ways of finding out whether a treatment sometimes causes harm

106

or some comparison treatment or placebo (the bottom row, whose total is **c+d**). Since the randomization would make them similar for all other features that would cause their deaths, you'd be pretty likely to judge any statistically significant increase in deaths among fenoterol recipients (cell **a**) as valid. Trouble is, if fenoterol causes only one extra death per 1000 users, you'd have to find an awfully big trial to show a clear excess among fenoterol-treated asthmatics. As it happens, if a drug causes an adverse reaction once per x patients who receive it (say, once per 1000), to be 95% certain to see at least one adverse reaction you need to follow 3x patients (in this example, 3000). For that reason, you usually can't find the most valid data on harm from individual randomized trials and if you can't find a systematic review with a large enough total number of patients to suffice, you'll have to work with non-experimental evidence.

The next most powerful design is also conducted along the rows of Table 3a4.2, but this time the groups of patients (called 'cohorts') who are (**a+b**) and are not (**c+d**) exposed to the treatment are formed not by random allocation, but by the decisions of clinicians and patients to have some of them ('exposed') receive the treatment and others ('unexposed') not receive it. These cohorts are then followed to determine which and how many of them develop the bad outcome (**a or c**). As you can see, there is no reason why these cohorts should be otherwise perfectly identical to each other and plenty of reason for them to be quite different (e.g. sicker patients who are more likely to have adverse outcomes might be more likely to be offered a 'last-ditch' treatment). Since there may be strong links between the prognosis of patients and the probability that they will be offered and accept a treatment (sometimes called 'confounding'), the analyses of these cohort analytic studies are difficult and often involve trying to correct for known confounders (such as disease severity) by statistical methods (all the way from simply comparing outcomes within patients with different degrees of severity to quite fancy multivariate analyses). But we can't adjust for what we don't yet know about the determinants of disease outcomes, so you have to be cautious in interpreting cohort studies.

And for rare or late complications of treatments, not even cohort studies are big enough and often you'll have to rely on studies conducted vertically in Table 3a4.2 by assembling cases (**a+c**) who already have the bad outcome, assembling a second group of 'controls' (**b+d**) who don't have the bad outcome and tracking back in their histories or records to determine the proportions of each group who were exposed to the suspect treatment (**a or b**): a case-control study. This is, in fact, what was done in trying to sort out the fenoterol problem: asthma deaths (cases) were compared with living asthma patients (controls) for their use of fenoterol and these comparisons were 'adjusted' for the severity of their asthma. The problem of confounding (of prognosis with exposure) is even worse in case-control studies than in cohort studies, for often it is impossible to measure the confounders among cases, even if they are known.* For this reason, case-control studies are viewed with even greater caution than cohort studies. Finally, you may find reports of one or a few patients who developed the bad outcome while under treatment (just cell **a**). If the outcome is unique and dramatic (phocomelia in children born to women who took thalidomide) case reports and case series may be enough, but usually they simply point to the need for the other types of studies.

As with other issues in clinical and health care, the best evidence on adverse effects will come from a systematic review of all the relevant studies and these should always be your primary targets when searching for the best external evidence. Systematic reviews of randomized trials or cohort studies may possess sufficiently large numbers of patients to identify even rare adverse effects. Whether appraising a systematic review or an individual study, you'll need to take into account how it assembled and assessed its members and now that you've learned how to recognize the sort of study you're reading, you can apply the guides in Table 3a4.1:

    1. From the foregoing discussion, it's clear why you want the report to describe clearly defined groups of

---

* Dead patients tell no tales and information about exposures to lethal treatments may perish with their victims.

patients, similar in all important ways other than exposure to the treatment (to get rid of confounders).
    2. Moreover, it makes sense that you should place greater confidence in reports of studies in which treatment exposures and clinical outcomes were measured the same ways in both groups (you'd not want one group studied more exhaustively than the other, because this would lead to reporting a greater occurrence of exposure or outcome in the more intensively studied group).
    3. Furthermore, in a report concluding that the treatment was innocent, you'd want the follow-up of study patients to have been complete and long enough for the bad effects to have had time to reveal themselves.
    4. Finally, you'd want to determine whether the association met at least some common-sense 'diagnostic tests for causation':
● you'd want to be sure that the exposure (say, use of a psychotropic drug) preceded the onset of the bad outcome (say, behavior ending in suicide), and wasn't just a 'marker' (say, of depression) that it was already underway;
● the validity of a claim that a treatment causes an adverse outcome receives a real boost when increasing doses or durations of the treatment are associated with increasing frequency or severity of the adverse outcome: a 'dose–response' effect;
● the validity of a claim is also boosted if there is documentation that the adverse effect decreased or disappeared when the treatment was withdrawn ('dechallenge') and worsened or reappeared when the treatment was reintroduced ('rechallenge');
● if you are fortunate enough to have found a systematic review of the question, you can determine whether the association of exposure to the suspect treatment and the adverse outcome is consistent from study to study. When it is, your confidence in the validity of the association deserves to increase;
● finally, it boosts your confidence when the association makes biological sense.

Table 3b1.1 Some pretest probabilities

Patient problem	Clinical setting	Target disorder	Pretest probability
Melena in a 50-year-old man who drinks 25 units of alcohol a week but has no stigmata of liver disease	Emergency room in North America	Varices	5%
		Benign ulcer	55%
		Gastritis	40%
Symptomless 60–69-year-olds	Primary care	Undiagnosed colon cancer: all patients positive family history	0.5% 1.5%
Symptomless Woman 30–39 y/o	Primary care	≥ 75% stenosis of one or more coronary arteries	0.3%
60–69 y/o			8%
Man 30–39 y/o			2%
60–69 y/o			12%
Non-anginal chest pain Woman 30–39 y/o			1%
60–69 y/o			19%
Man 30–39 y/o			5%
60–69 y/o			28%
Atypical angina Woman 30–39 y/o			4%
60–69 y/o			54%
Man 30–39 y/o			22%
60–69 y/o			67%
Typical angina pectoris Woman 30–39 y/o			26%
60–69 y/o			91%
Man 30–39 y/o			70%
60–69 y/o			94%
Symptomless 50 y/o with a solitary pulmonary nodule	Primary care	Cancer for any nodules For 3 cm nodules	50% 65%

To find more examples, and to nominate additions to the databank of pretest probabilities, refer to this textbook's Website at: http://cebm.jr2.ox.ac.uk/

Section 3b1

Is this evidence about a diagnostic test important?

In deciding whether the evidence about a diagnostic test is important, we will focus on a modern way of thinking about diagnosis that takes into account both components of evidence-based medicine: your individual clinical expertise and the best external evidence. The former is your prior assessment of diagnostic possibilities before you do the test ('prior or pretest probabilities') and the latter is the ability of the test to distinguish patients with and without the target disorder (both the oldfashioned concepts of sensitivity and specificity and the newfangled and more powerful ideas around likelihood ratios). We'll show you how to combine these two elements of EBM to refine your estimates of the target disorder ('posterior or post-test probabilities') and make the diagnosis. Diagnostic tests that produce big changes from pretest to post-test probabilities are important and likely to be useful to you in your practice.

Where do these pretest probabilities come from? Usually they are derived from your own accumulating clinical experience, specific for the setting in which you work and the sorts of patients you see. As a result, pretest probabilities for the same target disorder can vary widely between and within countries and between primary, secondary and tertiary care. We have summarized some published pretest probabilities in Table 3b1.1 and more are available from our Website.

Suppose that you're working up a patient with anemia and think that the probability that they have iron deficiency anemia is 50%; that is, the odds are about 50–50 that it's due to iron deficiency. When you present the patient to your boss, you ask for an educational prescription to determine the usefulness of performing a serum ferritin on your patient as a means of detecting iron deficiency anemia. Suppose further that, in filling your prescription, you find a systematic

If the report fails to meet the first three minimum standards, you're better off abandoning it and continuing your search. On the other hand, if you're satisfied that the report meets these minimum guides, you can decide whether the relation between exposure and outcome is strong and convincing enough for you to need to do something about it and that's discussed in Section 3b4.

Further reading

Levine M, Walter S D, Lee H, Haines T, Holbrook A, Moyer V for the Evidence-Based Medicine Working Group. Users' guides to the medical literature: IV. How to use an article about harm. JAMA 1994; 271: 1615–19.

Evidence-based Medicine

review of several studies of this diagnostic test (evaluated against the reference standard of a bone marrow stain for iron), decide that it is valid (based on the guides in Tables 3a3.2 and 3a1.1), and find their results as shown in Table 3b1.2. By the time you've tracked down and studied the external evidence, your patient's serum ferritin comes back at 60 mmol/L. How should you put all this together?

As you can see from Table 3b1.2, your patient's result places them in the top row of the table, either in cell **a** or cell **b**. From that fact you would conclude several things: first, you'd note that 90% of patients with iron deficiency have serum ferritins in the same range as your patient, (**a/(a+c)**), and that property, the proportion of patients with the target disorder who have positive test results, is called sensitivity.

Table 3b1.2 Results of a systematic review of serum ferritin as a diagnostic test for iron deficiency anemia

Diagnostic test result (serum ferritin)	Target disorder (iron deficiency anemia)		Totals
	Present	Absent	
Positive (<65 mmol/L)	731 (a)	270 (b)	1001 (a+b)
Negative (≥65 mmol/L)	78 (c)	1500 (d)	1578 (c+d)
Totals	809 (a+c)	1770 (b+d)	2579 (a+b+c+d)

Sensitivity = **a/(a+c)** = 731/809 = 90%
Specificity = **d/(b+d)** = 1500/1770 = 85%
LR+ = sens/(1-spec) = 90%/15% = 6
LR- = (1-sens)/spec = 10%/85% = 0.12
Positive predictive value = **a/(a+b)** = 731/1001 = 73%
Negative predictive value = **d/(c+d)** = 1500/1578 = 95%
Prevalence = **(a+c)/(a+b+c+d)** = prevalence/((1-prevalence) = 809/2579 = 32%
Pretest odds = prevalence/((1-prevalence) = 31%/69% = 0.45
Post-test odds = pretest odds × likelihood ratio
Post-test probability = post-test odds/(post-test odds +1)

And you might also note that only 15% of patients with other causes for their anemia have results in the same range as your patient,* which means that your patient's result would be about six times as likely (90% / 15%) to be seen in someone with, as opposed to someone without, iron deficiency anemia and that's called the likelihood ratio for a positive test result. Furthermore, since you thought ahead of time (before you had the result of the serum ferritin) that your patient's odds of iron deficiency were 50–50, that's called a pretest odds of 1:1 and, as you can see from the formulae towards the bottom of Table 3b1.2, you can multiply that pretest odds of 1 by the likelihood ratio of 6 to get the post-test odds of iron deficiency anemia after the test: 1×6 = 6. Since, like most clinicians, you may be more comfortable thinking in terms of probabilities than odds, this post-test odds of 6:1 converts (as you can see at the bottom of Table 3b1.2) to a post-test probability of 6/(6+1) = 6/7 = 86%. So it looks like you've made the diagnosis and this diagnostic test looks worthwhile.

(To check yourself out on these calculations, try the same ferritin result for a patient who, like those in the table, has a pretest odds of 0.47;† you'll know you did it right if you wind up with an answer identical to its equivalent, the positive predictive value.)

Extremely high values of sensitivity and specificity are useful, but not for the reasons you may think.‡ When a test has a very high sensitivity (such as the loss of retinal vein pulsation in increased intracranial pressure), a negative result (the presence of pulsation) effectively rules out the diagnosis (of raised intracranial pressure) and one of our clinical clerks suggested that we apply the mnemonic SnNout to such findings (when a sign has a high Sensitivity, a Negative result

---

* The complement of this proportion is called specificity and it describes the proportion of patients who do not have the target disorder who have negative or normal test results, **d/(b+d)**.
† The post-test odds are 0.45 × 6 = 2.7 and the post-test probability is 2.7/3.7 = 73%. Note that this is identical to the positive predictive value.
‡ On first encounter, most learners think that tests with high sensitivity rule in diagnoses and tests with high specificity rule them out; the reverse is the case.

rules *out* the diagnosis). Similarly, when a sign has a very high specificity (such as a fluid wave for ascites), a positive result effectively rules in the diagnosis (of ascites); not surprisingly, our clinical clerks call such a finding a SpPin (when a sign has a high Specificity, a Positive result rules in the diagnosis). We've listed some SpPins and SnNouts in Table 3b1.3 and have generated a longer list on our Website.

Although the serum ferritin determination looks impressive when viewed in terms of its sensitivity (90%) and specificity (85%), the newer way of expressing its accuracy with likelihood ratios reveals its even greater power and, in this particular example, shows how we can be misled by the fact that the old sensitivity–specificity approach restricts us to just two levels (positive and negative) of the test result. Most test results, like serum ferritin, can be divided into several levels and in Table 3b1.4 we show you a particularly useful way of dividing test results into five levels. When this is done, one extreme level of the test result can be shown to rule in the diagnosis and in this case you can SpPin 59% of the patients with iron deficiency anemia, despite the unimpressive sensitivity (59%) that would have been achieved if the ferritin results had been split at this level. Likelihood ratios of 10 or more, when applied to pretest probabilities of 33% or more (.33/.67 = pretest odds of 0.5) will generate post-test probabilities of 5/6 = 83% or more. Moreover, the other extreme level can SnNout 75% of those who do not have iron deficiency anemia (again despite a not very impressive specificity of 75%). Likelihood ratios of 0.1 or less, when applied to pretest probabilities of 33% or less (.33/.67 = pretest odds of 0.5) will generate post-test probabilities of 0.05/1.05 = 5% or less. Two other intermediate levels can move a 50% prior probability (pretest odds of 1:1) to the useful but not usually diagnostic post-test probabilities of 4.8/5.8 = 83% and 0.39/1.39 = 28%. And one indeterminate level in the middle (containing about 10% of both sorts of patients) can be seen to be uninformative, with a likelihood ratio of 1. We've shown the effects of these sorts of likelihood ratios on these sorts of pretest probabilities in Table 3b1.5.

Table 3b1.3 Some SpPins and SnNouts

Target disorder	SpPin (& specificity) [presence rules in the target disorder]	SnNout (& sensitivity) [absence rules out the target disorder]
Ascites (by imaging or tap)*	Fluid wave (92%)	History of ankle swelling (93%)
Pleural effusion†	Auscultatory percussion note loud and sharp (100%)	Auscultatory percussion note soft and/or dull (96%)
Increased intracranial pressure (by CAT scan or direct measurement)‡		Loss of spontaneous retinal vein pulsation (100%)
Cancer as a cause of lower back pain (by further investigation)§		Age >50 or cancer history or unexplained weight loss or failure of conservative therapy (100%)
Sinusitis (by further investigation)¶		Maxillary toothache or purulent nasal secretion or poor response to nasal decongestants or abnormal transillumination or history of coloured nasal discharge
Alcohol abuse or dependency**	Yes to ≥3 of the CAGE questions (99.8%)	
Splenomegaly (by imaging)††	Positive percussion (Nixon method) and palpation	
Non-urgent cause for dizziness‡‡	Positive head-hanging test and either vertigo or vomiting (94%)	

To find more examples, and to nominate additions to the databank of SpPins and SnNouts, refer to this textbook's Website at: http://cebm.jr2.ox.ac.uk/
* JAMA 1992; 267: 2645–8.
† J Gen Int Med 1994; 9: 71–4.
‡ Arch Neurol 1978; 35: 37–40.
§ JAMA 1992; 268: 760–5.
¶ JAMA 1993; 270: 1242–6.
** Amer J Med 1987; 82: 231–5.
†† JAMA 1993; 270: 2218–21.
‡‡ JAMA 1994; 271: 385–8.

Table 3b1.4 The usefulness of five levels of a diagnostic test result

Diagnostic test result	Serum ferritin (mmol/L)	Target disorder present Number	%	Target disorder absent Number	%	Likelihood ratio	Diagnostic impact
Very positive	<15	474	59%	20	1.1%	52	Rule in SpPin
Moderately positive	15–34	175	22%	79	4.5%	4.8	intermediate high
Neutral	35–64	82	10%	171	10%	1	indeterminate
Moderately negative	65–94	30	3.7%	168	9.5%	0.39	intermediate low
Extremely negative	≥95	48	5.9%	1332	75%	0.08	Rule out SnNout
		809	100%	1770	100%		

Table 3b1.5 Some post-test probabilities generated by five levels of a diagnostic test result

Likelihood ratio	Post-test probability of the target disorder for different pretest probabilities						Diagnostic impact
	Pre-test 5%	Pre-test 10%	Pre-test 20%	Pre-test 30%	Pre-test 50%	Pre-test 70%	
Very positive 10	34%	53%	71%	81%	91%	96%	Rule in SpPin
Moderately positive 3	14%	25%	43%	56%	75%	88%	Intermediate high
Neutral 1	5%	10%	20%	30%	50%	70%	Indeterminate
Moderately negative 0.3	1.5%	3.2%	7%	11%	23%	41%	Intermediate low
Extremely negative 0.1	0.5%	1%	2.5%	4%	9%	19%	Rule out SnNout

Evidence-based Medicine

123

124

125

Finally, there's an easier way of manipulating all these probability↔odds calculations and a nomogram for doing so appears as Figure 3b1.1 and in the pocket cards that come with this book. You can check out your understanding of this nomogram by replicating the results in Table 3b1.5.

To your surprise (we reckon!) your patient's test result generates an indeterminate likelihood ratio of only 1 and the test which you thought might be very useful, based on the sensitivity and specificity way of looking at things, really hasn't been helpful in moving you toward the diagnosis, so you'll have to think about other tests (including perhaps the reference standard of a bone marrow examination) to sort this out.

More and more reports of diagnostic tests are providing multilevel likelihood ratios as measures of their accuracy. When they only report sensitivity and specificity, you can sometimes find a table with more levels and generate your own set of likelihood ratios or you can find a scatter plot (of test results versus diagnoses) that is good enough for you to be able to split into levels. Or, if all you have is sensitivity and specificity, you can generate likelihood ratios from them by reference to the formulae in Table 3b1.2 (the likelihood ratio for a positive test result = LR+ = sensitivity/[1-specificity] and the likelihood ratio for a negative test result = LR− = [1-sensitivity]/specificity).

Some reports into the accuracy of diagnostic tests go beyond even likelihood ratios and one of them deserves mention here. This extension considers multiple diagnostic tests as a cluster or sequence of tests for a given target disorder. These multiple results can be presented in different ways, either as clusters of positive/negative results or as multivariate scores, and in either case they can be ranked and handled just like other multilevel likelihood ratios.

In any event, having decided that a diagnostic test produces important changes from pretest to post-test probabilities, you might want to study the final issue, described in Section 4.1, of how to integrate the results of this critical appraisal with your individual clinical expertise and apply the results

to your own patient (but if you jumped to this second step without first determining whether the evidence about this diagnostic test was valid, you'd better go back to Section 3a1 first!).

Further reading

Sackett D L, Haynes R B, Guyatt G H, Tugwell P. Clinical epidemiology: a basic science for clinical medicine, 2nd edn. Little, Brown, Boston, 1991. Chapter 4 (for interpreting diagnostic tests).

Jaeschke R, Guyatt G H, Sackett D L for the Evidence-Based Medicine Working Group. Users' guides to the medical literature. VI. How to use an article about a diagnostic test. A. Are the results of the study valid? JAMA 1994; 271: 389–91. B. What are the results and will they help me in caring for my patients? JAMA 1994; 271: 703–7.

Nomogram for interpreting diagnostic test result

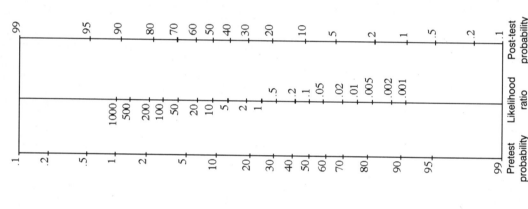

Figure 3b1.1 A likelihood ratio nomogram. Adapted from Fagan T J 1975 Nomogram for Bayes's Theorem (c). New England Journal of Medicine 293: 257

Section 3b2

Is this evidence about prognosis important?

Guides for making this decision appear in Table 3b2.1. First, how likely are the outcomes over time? Diseases usually have more than a single outcome of interest and these can occur in several combinations and at different times following the onset of the disease. Thus, for each important disease outcome, you should examine the article to see how likely each of these outcomes is over time. Typically they are reported as percentage survival at a particular point in time (such as 1-year or 5-year survival rates) and as survival curves of various kinds. Another form of result, common in cancer studies, is the median survival, indicating the length of follow-up by which 50% of the study sample have died. The more numerous the outcome possibilities and the more variable the timing of these outcomes are, the more complex such results can be.

Figure 3b2.1 illustrates some different patterns of prognosis, each leading to different conclusions about prognosis. They are presented in the most frequent format used to describe prognosis, a survival curve that depicts, at each point in time, the proportion (often expressed as a %) of the original study population who have NOT yet had an outcome event.* In panel A, virtually no patients have had events by the end of the study, so either the prognosis is very good (in which case the study is very useful to you) or the study is too short (in which case it's not very useful!). Panels B, C and D depict a serious disease, with only

---

* How such survival curves are constructed is not described in detail in this book, so don't look for it! In brief, it is done by some clever methods that combine the results from patients who have been followed for just short periods of time as well as long ones and who have had outcomes occur early, late or not at all. Often the strategy used here is a 'life table' method, if you want to look it up.

Table 3b2.1 Is this evidence about prognosis important?

1. How likely are the outcomes over time?
2. How precise are the prognostic estimates?

20% of patients surviving at 1 year; you could tell such patients, then, that their chances of surviving for a year are 20%. Note, however, that the shapes of these curves are quite different, so that the median survival (by which time half of them have succumbed) is 9 months for the disorder described in panel B but only 3 months for the disorder described in panel C. The survival pattern is a steady, uniform decline only in panel D and we hope you can see why the best answer to 'How much time have I got, doc?' often is the time at which half the study patients have died (or suffered some other event of interest); this is called the median survival.

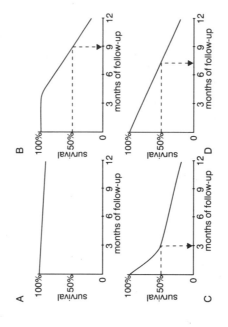

Figure 3b2.1 Prognosis shown as survival curves. Panel A: Good prognosis (or too short a study!). Panel B: Good prognosis early, then worsening, with a median survival of 9 months. Panel C: Bad prognosis early, then better, with a median survival of 3 months. Panel D: Steady prognosis, with a median survival of 6 months

---

The second guide asks you to consider how precise the prognostic statements are. As we mentioned in Section 3a2, investigators study prognosis in a sample of diseased patients, not in the whole population of everyone who has ever had the disease. Purely by the play of chance, then, the identical study done 100 times over with different samples from that same whole population would yield differing results. In deciding whether these prognostic results are important, then, you will need some means of judging just how much these results could vary by chance alone, that is, the precision of the results. This is best done with the 95% confidence interval:* in those 100 repetitions of the identical study with different samples, 95 would be within a calculable distance of the true prognosis (some lower and some higher). For example, an article on the prognosis of first strokes among 675 patients reported a case-fatality rate of 20% in the first month, with the 95% confidence interval of 17–23%; that interval is pretty narrow and if the report was valid, it looks important as well. If, on the other hand, that 20% was based on just 20 patients, the 95% confidence interval on death in the first month would run from 2% to 38% and that is so wide (almost 20-fold) that you couldn't regard the result as important and potentially useful to you. The text, tables or graphs should tell you the confidence interval for the prognosis and you can decide whether it is too big for you to trust it.

That completes your critical appraisal of evidence about prognosis. If you decide that the evidence you've found is both valid and important, you could go to Section 2 of Chapter 4 (page 164) and decide whether and how to apply it to your patient.

---

* We describe the confidence interval in the Appendix. In this case, the confidence interval on a prognosis (expressed as a decimal) is the observed result plus or minus 1.96 times the square root of {[(the observed result) × (1 – the observed result)] / sample size}. So, for the original study 20% = 0.2 and the confidence interval becomes 0.2 +/– 1.96 times the square root of {[(0.2) × (0.8)]/675} or 0.2 +/– 0.03 or 17–23%. As a check on your understanding, you can see if you can calculate the confidence interval when the sample is just 40 stroke patients.

Further reading

Laupacis A, Wells G, Richardson W S, Tugwell P for the Evidence-Based Medicine Working Group. Users' guides to the medical literature. V. How to use an article about prognosis. JAMA 1994; 272: 234–7.

Section 3b3

Is this evidence about a treatment important?

This section will help you determine the size and potential benefits of the effects of the treatment described in a report, whether you've decided (from the previous section) that the report is valid or whether you start here. Because our primary perspective in this book is the individual clinician, the main measure we will show you how to develop and use is the number of patients a clinician needs to treat in order to prevent one additional adverse outcome (NNT) and along the way we will show you both the absolute risk reduction (ARR) and relative risk reduction (RRR) in the occurrence of adverse outcomes achieved by active therapy. We'll also introduce you to the bare bones of assessing the results of an economic analysis, a more complex method that we employ in determining the effects of therapy when we are taking the broader perspective (usually in collaboration with health managers) of deciding how groups of patients, or society as a whole, should be provided or offered treatments in the way that best uses scarce resources such as hospital beds, drugs, operating time, clinicians and money. Finally, we'll give you a brief description of how evidence on the effects of therapy can be formulated into a clinical decision analysis.

In Section 3 of Chapter 4, we'll show you how to extrapolate the measures from each of these three approaches to individual patients, in order to answer the question: Can I apply these results to my patient?

Is the evidence from this randomized trial important?

Introducing some measures of the effects of therapy

Knowing whether you should be impressed with the results of a valid therapeutic trial requires two steps: first, finding the

most useful clinical expression of these results (or converting data from the report into this most useful expression); and second, comparing those results with the results of other treatments for other conditions. We'll take these one at a time.

The relative risk reduction (RRR)

The Diabetes Control and Complications Trial into the effect of intensive diabetes therapy on the development and progression of neuropathy, which we've summarized in Table 3b3.1, confirmed neuropathy occurred among 9.6% of patients randomized to usual care (1–2 insulin injections/day to prevent glycemic symptoms; we'll call that the control event rate or CER) and 2.8% (we'll call that the experimental event rate or EER) among patients randomized to intensive therapy (insulin pump or =>3 injections per day).

This difference was statistically highly significant, but how might this treatment effect be expressed in terms of its clinical significance? The traditional measure of this effect is the proportional or 'relative' risk reduction (abbreviated RRR in our journal), calculated as (CER–EER)/CER. In this example, the RRR is (9.6% – 2.8%) / 9.6% or 71%; intensive therapy reduced the risk of developing neuropathy by 71%.

Why not confine our description of the clinical significance of this result to the relative risk reduction (RRR)? The reason is that the RRR fails to discriminate huge absolute treatment effects (10 times those observed in this trial) from trivial ones (one ten-thousandth of those observed here). For example, if the rates of neuropathy were 10 times those observed in this trial (the 'high hypothetical case' in Table 3b3.1), and a whopping 96% of control patients and 28% of intensively treated patients developed neuropathy, the relative risk reduction would remain unchanged: RRR = (96% – 28%) / 96% or 71%. And if a trivial 0.00096% of control and 0.00028% of intensively treated patients developed neuropathy (the 'low hypothetical case' in Table 3b3.1), the relative risk reduction is as before: RRR still = (0.00096% − 0.00028%) / 0.00096 = 71%! This is because the relative risk reduction discards the underlying susceptibility (or 'baseline risk') of patients entering randomized trials; as a result, the relative risk reduction cannot discriminate huge risks and benefits from small ones.

The absolute risk reduction (ARR)

In contrast to these non-discriminating relative risk reductions, the absolute difference in the rates of neuropathy between control and experimental patients (CER−EER) clearly does discriminate between these extremes and this measure is called the absolute risk reduction or ARR. In the trial, the ARR or (CER−EER) = 9.6% − 2.8% = 6.8%; in the high hypothetical case, where 96% of control patients and 28% of intensively treated patients developed neuropathy, the ARR = 96% − 28% = 68% and in the low hypothetical case in which a trivial 0.00096% of control and 0.00028% of intensively treated patients developed neuropathy, the ARR = 0.00096% − 0.00028% = 0.00068%. These absolute risk reductions retain the underlying susceptibility of patients and provide more complete information than relative risk reductions. And when treatment increases the occurrence of some good event (rather than decreasing the occurrence of some bad event) we can generate an absolute risk increase or ARI. But, unlike relative risk reductions (RRRs), absolute risk reductions and increases (ARRs and ARIs) are difficult to remember and don't slip easily off the tongue at the bedside (lots of clinicians become queasy with numbers less than 1.0).

The number of patients that need to be treated (NNT) to prevent one bad outcome

If, however, we divide the absolute risk reduction into 1 (that is, if we 'invert' the ARR or 'take its reciprocal' so that it becomes 1/ARR), we generate a very useful number, for it represents the number of patients we need to treat (NNT) with the experimental therapy in order to prevent one of them from developing the bad outcome.* In this case, we would generate the number of diabetics we would need to treat with the intensive regimen in order to prevent one of them from developing neuropathy. In the trial, the NNT is 1/ARR or 1/6.8% or 14.7; we usually round that number upwards (in this case, to 15) and we now can say that for every 15 patients who are treated with the more intensive insulin regimen, one will be prevented from developing diabetic neuropathy.

Is this a large or a small number of patients that need to be treated to prevent one bad outcome? Now we're ready to pursue that second step in deciding whether to be impressed with the valid results of a therapeutic trial. Like many important matters in medicine, the answer has to do with clinical significance, not statistical significance. This NNT of 15 certainly is far smaller than the number of patients we'd need to treat in the extremely low hypothetical example, in which 1/ARR becomes 1/(0.00068%) or an NNT of more than 147 000, a figure so vast that we can't imagine anyone judging that it was worth the effort. We can get a better idea by comparing this NNT of 15 with that for other interventions we are familiar with in medicine.

In doing so, we add the additional dimension of the duration of therapy: in the diabetes trial treatment went on for an average of 6.5 years, meaning that we need to treat about 15 diabetics for about 6.5 years with an intensive insulin regimen to prevent one of them from developing neuropathy. How does this compare with other treatments, over other durations, for other conditions? We show some of them (with the event rates appearing as decimals rather than percents) in Table 3b3.2. Beginning on an optimistic note, we need to treat only about 20 chest pain patients who appear to be having heart attacks with streptokinase and aspirin to save a life at 5 weeks. On the other hand, we need to treat about 70 elderly hypertensives for 5 years with antihypertensive drugs

---

* Similarly, 1/ARI tells us how many individuals we need to treat to cause one additional good outcome.

Table 3b3.1 Clinically useful measures of the effects of treatment

The occurrence of neuropathy	Event rates (diabetic neuropathy)		Relative risk reduction RRR = CER−EER / CER	Absolute risk reduction ARR = (CER−EER)	Number needed to be treated (to prevent one event) NNT = 1/ARR
	Usual insulin regimen (CER)	Intensive insulin regimen (EER)			
In the actual trial	9.6%	2.8%	$\frac{9.6\%-2.8\%}{9.6\%}$ = 71%	9.6% − 2.8% = 6.8%	$\frac{1}{6.8\%}$ = 14.7 or 15
High hypothetical case A	96%	28%	$\frac{96\%-28\%}{96\%}$ = 71%	(96%−28%) = 68%	$\frac{1}{68\%}$ = 1.47 or 2
Low hypothetical case B	0.00096%	0.00028%	$\frac{(0.00096\%-0.00028\%)}{(0.00096\%)}$ = 71%	(0.00096% −0.00028%) = 0.00068%	$\frac{1}{0.00068\%}$ = 147 000

to save one life, about 100 men with no evidence of coronary heart disease for 5 years with aspirin to prevent one heart attack and about 10 patients with symptomatic moderate to severe carotid artery stenosis with endarterectomy to prevent one major or fatal stroke over the following 2 years.

We think that the 'number needed to be treated' (NNT) to prevent one event is the most useful measure of the clinical effort we and our patients must expend in order to help them avoid bad outcomes to their illnesses. Note, however, that this is a measure with real meaning for clinicians, but not for individual patients (who are interested in Ns of 1, not NNTs). Furthermore, because we are focusing here on the magnitude of the treatment effect, rather than on the probability that we have drawn a false-positive conclusion that the treatment is at all effective (when it is not), we should employ confidence intervals around the NNT, specifying the 'limits' within which we can confidently state the true NNT lies (95% of the time), rather than focus just on p-values. Readers who want to brush up on confidence intervals can refer to the Appendix.

Since we are interested in the risks as well as the benefits of treatments, we can generate a parallel 'number needed to harm' or NNH to express the downside of therapy. For example, if anticoagulation carries an annual risk of major bleeding of 2%, the NNH is 1/2% = 50.

Overviews and metaanalyses often provide NNTs, but sometimes only report odds ratios. The latter are not the same as RRRs and can be converted into RRRs on when you know the patient's expected event rate (PEER) by using the formula:

$$NNT = \frac{1 - [PEER \times (1 - OR)]}{(1 - PEER) \times PEER \times (1 - OR)}$$

To help you 'translate' odds ratios to NNTs (without having to crank through this formula), we've summarized several of them in Table 3b3.3.

The NNT from the published report, in light of your own clinical expertise and compared with those in Table 3b3.2, will give you an idea of whether the treatment is potentially

* Ann Intern Med 1995;122:561-8. EBM 1995;1:9.
† Diabetes Res Clin Pract 1995;28:103-17
‡ Lancet 1988;2:349-60.
§ JAMA 1967;202:116-22.
¶ BMJ 1985;291:97-104.
** N Engl J Med 1995;333:1184-9. EBM 1996;1:87.
†† Lancet 1995;345:1455-63. EBM 1996;1:44.
‡‡ Lancet 1993;341:973-8.
§§ N Engl J Med 1991;325:445-53.
¶¶ Am J Obstet Gynecol 1995;173:322-35. EBM 1996;1:92.

To find more examples, and to nominate additions to the databank of NNTs, refer to this textbook's Web Page at: http://cebm.jr2.ox.ac.uk/

Table 3b3.2 Some NNTs for different treatments

Condition or disorder	Intervention	Events being prevented	Event Rates		Duration of follow-up	NNT to prevent one additional event
			Control Event Rate CER	Experimental Event Rate EER		
Diabetes (IDDM)*	Intensive insulin regimens	Diabetic neuropathy	0.096	0.028	6.5 years	15
Diabetes (NIDDM)†	Intensive insulin regimens	Worse diabetic retinopathy	0.38	0.13	6 years	4
		Nephropathy	0.30	0.10		5
Acute myocardial infarction‡	Streptokinase and Aspirin	Death at 5 weeks	0.134	0.081	5 weeks	19
		Death at 2 years	0.216	0.174	2 years	24
Diastolic blood pressure 115-129 mm Hg§	Antihypertensive drugs	Death, stroke or myocardial infarction	0.1286	0.0137	1.5 years	3
Diastolic blood pressure 90-109 mm Hg¶	Antihypertensive drugs	Death, stroke or myocardial infarction	0.0545	0.0467	5.5 years	128
Independent elderly people**	Comprehensive geriatric home assessment	Long-term nursing home admission	0.10	0.04	3 years	17
Pregnant women with eclampsia††	iv MgSO₄ (vs. diazepam)	Recurrent convulsion	0.279	0.132	hours	7
Healthy women ages 50-69‡‡	Breast examination plus mammography	Death from breast cancer	0.00345	0.00252	9 years	1075
Symptomatic high-grade carotid artery stenosis§§	Carotid endarterectomy	Major stroke or death	0.181	0.08	2 years	10
Preterm babies¶¶	Antenatal corticosteroids	Respiratory distress syndrome	0.23	0.13	days	11

Evidence-based Medicine

Table 3b3.3 Translating odds ratios to NNTs

		Odds ratio			
		0.9	0.8	0.7	0.6	0.5
Patient's	.05	209*	104	69	52	41†
expected	.10	110	54	36	27	21
event	.20	61	30	20	14	11
rate	.30	46	22	14	10	8
(PEER)	.40	40	19	12	9	7
	.50	38	18	11	8	6
	.70	44	20	13	9	6
	.90	101‡	46	27	18	12§

The numbers in the body of the table are the NNTs for the corresponding odds ratios at that particular patient's expected event rate (PEER).
* The relative risk reduction (RRR) here is 49%.
† The RRR here is 10%.
‡ The RRR here is 1%.
§ The RRR here is 9%.

useful for your patient. In the next chapter, we will show you a very simple way to find out whether this potential is met for your individual patient.

tive to untreated patients, calculated as $[a/(a+b)]/[c/(c+d)]$. Thus, if 1000 patients receive a treatment and 20 of them have an adverse outcome, **a**=20 and **a/(a+b)** = 20/1000 = 2%; and if just two of 1000 patients with the same condition but receiving a different treatment suffered this adverse outcome, **c**=2 and **c/(c+d)** = 2/1000 = 0.2% and the relative risk = 2%/0.2% or 10. That is, patients receiving the suspect treatment were 10 times as likely to suffer the adverse outcome as patients treated some other way.

In a case-control study, where patients with and without the adverse outcome are selected and tracked backward to their prior treatments, strength (which in this case is called the odds ratio) can only be indirectly estimated as **ad/bc**. For example, if 100 cases of the adverse outcome are assembled and it is discovered that 90 of them had received the suspect treatment, **a**=90 and **c**=10; if 100 control patients, free of the adverse outcome, are also assembled and it is discovered that only 45 of them received the suspect treatment, **b**=45 and **d**=55, and the relative odds = **ad/bc** = (90×55)/(45×10) = 11. That is, patients receiving the suspect treatment are 11 times as likely to suffer the adverse event as patients treated some other way.

Section 3b4

Is this evidence about harm important?

The main measure that indicates whether valid evidence that a treatment harms some patients is also impressive (and potentially useful clinically) is the strength of the association between receiving the treatment and suffering the adverse effect. Strength here means the risk or odds of the adverse effect with, as opposed to without, exposure to the treatment; the higher the risk or odds, the greater the strength and the more you should be impressed with it.

Different tactics for estimating the strength of association are used in different types of studies and these are shown in Table 3b4.1. In the randomized trial and cohort study, patients who were and were not exposed to the treatment are carefully followed up to find out whether they develop the adverse outcome, with the risk in the treated patients, rela-

Table 3b4.1 Different ways of calculating the strength of an association between a treatment and subsequent adverse outcomes

		Adverse outcome		Totals
		Present (Case)	Absent (Control)	
Exposed to the treatment	Yes (Cohort)	a	b	a+b
	No (Cohort)	c	d	c+d
	Totals	a+c	b+d	a+b+c+d

In a randomized trial or cohort study: relative risk = RR = $[a/(a+b)]/[c/(c+d)]$
In a case-control study: relative odds = RO = **ad/bc**

How big should relative risks and relative odds become before you should be impressed with them? This question has two answers. First, you'd like to be confident that the relative risk (RR) or relative odds (RO) is really greater than 1 (when RR or RO = 1, the adverse outcome is no greater with than without exposure to the suspect treatment). So, as before, you'd want to be sure that the entire confidence interval remains within a clinically important range of RR or RO. Second, the size of the 'impressive' RR or RO depends on the type of study from which it is generated. Because of the biases we described in case-control studies, you'd want to be sure that the RO was greater than that which could arise from bias alone and you might not want to become impressed with their ROs until they reach 4 or more (some of our colleagues would relax these guides for a serious adverse effect and set them even higher for a trivial one). Since cohort studies are less subject to bias, you might be impressed with RRs of 3 or more in them. And because randomized trials are relatively free of bias, any RR whose confidence interval excludes 1 is impressive and warrants further consideration.

Having decided that you are impressed with both the validity and the strength of the relationship between the suspect treatment and the adverse outcome, you then need to translate this into some measure of the impact of changing your treatment strategy on the occurrence of the adverse outcome and decide whether it is worth the effort required to achieve it. The measures we've employed up to now, the RR and OR, don't provide this information very well and you need to return to the concept of the NNT. In this case you are concerned about a bad outcome and you might want to revise the term to the 'number of patients needed to be treated to produce one episode of harm' or NNH. Our reason for doing this is that the RR and OR are fine for determining whether the link to harm was true, but don't tell us whether the link was clinically important. For example, a cohort study showed that NSAIDS can cause gastrointestinal bleeding and the confidence interval on the relative risk for this adverse outcome included 2. A randomized trial showed that the antiarrhythmic drugs encainide and flecainide can cause death and the confidence interval on the relative risk for this adverse outcome also included 2. But the absolute increase in the risk of bleeding in the former study was small, at about 0.05%, which translates to an NNH of 2000 to cause one more GI bleed, whereas the absolute increase in the risk of death in the latter trial was 4.7% or an NNH of 21 to cause one additional death! Clearly, similar RRs or ORs can lead to very different NNHs and you need the latter as well as the former to make your clinical decision about your patient.

That final step of integrating this external evidence with your clinical expertise is discussed in Section 4.4.

Further reading

Levine M, Walter S D, Lee H, Haines T, Holbrook A, Moyer V for the Evidence-Based Medicine Working Group. Users' guides to the medical literature: IV. How to use an article about harm. JAMA 1994; 271: 1615–19.

Section 4.1

Can you apply this valid, important evidence about a diagnostic test in caring for your patient?

Having found a valid systematic review or individual report about a diagnostic test and decided that its accuracy is sufficiently high to be useful, how do you integrate it with your individual clinical expertise and apply it to your patient?

There are three questions whose answers dictate this determination, summarized in Table 4.1.1. First, is the diagnostic test available, affordable, accurate and precise in your setting? You obviously can't order a test that's not available but even if it is, you may want to check around to be sure that it's performed and interpreted in a competent, reproducible fashion and that its potential consequences (see below) justify its cost. Moreover, diagnostic tests often behave differently among different subsets of patients, generating higher likelihood ratios in later stages of florid disease and lower likelihood ratios in early, mild stages. This is another reason why multilevel likelihood ratios are helpful, as there are at least theoretical reasons why they should suffer less distortion from this cause. Finally, it is known that at least some diagnostic tests based on symptoms or signs lose power as patients move from primary care to secondary and tertiary care. Reference back to Table 3b1.1 can show you why: if patients are referred onward in part because of symptoms, their primary care clinicians will be sending along patients in both cells **a** and **b** and subsequent evaluations of the accuracy of their symptoms will tend to show falling specificity due to the referral of patients with false-positive findings. If you think that any of these factors may be operating, you can try out what you judge to be clinically sensible variations in the likelihood ratios for your test result and see whether the results alter your post-test probabilities in a way that changes your diagnosis (the short-hand term for this sort of exploration is 'sensitivity analysis').

The second question you need to answer is whether you can generate a clinically sensible estimate of your patient's pretest probability. Sometimes you've actually got the data on pretest probabilities from your practice or institution. That's wonderful when it exists and constitutes a reason to consider keeping some records on the pretest probabilities for important diagnoses you eventually make for the specific presenting complaints in which you'd consider this sort of diagnostic test. Sometimes, you've had enough experience both to be able to make this estimation based on your own experience and to know how your estimate can be distorted by your last case (either way, depending on whether you ruled in or ruled out the diagnosis), your most dramatic or embarrassing case (usually this either distorts your pretest odds upwards or makes you reluctant to quit testing until the post-test odds are vanishingly small) or by whether you are an expert in the evaluation or care of patients with this diagnosis (which usually makes you reluctant to miss one).

Early in your career or when you haven't previously encountered this diagnostic situation, you'll be less certain about your patient's pretest probability. When that happens, you can try one or more of the following. First, if

Table 4.1.1 Questions to answer in applying a valid diagnostic test to an individual patient

1. Is the diagnostic test available, affordable, accurate and precise in your setting?
2. Can you generate a clinically sensible estimate of your patient's pretest probability:
   - from practice data?
   - from personal experience?
   - from the report itself?
   - from clinical speculation?
3. Will the resulting post-test probabilities affect your management and help your patient?
   - Could it move you across a test-treatment threshold?
   - Would your patient be a willing partner in carrying it out?
   - Would the consequences of the test help your patient reach their goals in all this?

your setting and patient closely resemble those that appeared in the report, you can use its pretest probability. Or if your patient is a bit different from those in the study, you can use its pretest probability as a starting point and again set off on a sensitivity analysis using clinically sensible variations in pretest probabilities and determining their impact on the test's usefulness. As before, the issue here is not whether your patient is exactly like those in the report, but whether they are so different that the report is of no help in making the diagnosis. Finally, you may simply go straight to a sensitivity analysis in which you plug the likelihood ratios from your report into a range of sensible pretest probabilities and see what the likely range of post-test probabilities will be (perhaps using the entries in Table 3b1.4 on page 124 to help you).

The final question you need to answer is: Will the resulting post-test probabilities affect your management and help your patient? The elements of this answer are three. First, could its results move you across some threshold that would cause you to stop all further testing? Two thresholds should be borne in mind. If the diagnostic test was negative or generated a likelihood ratio well below 1.0, the post-test probability might become so low that you would abandon the diagnosis it was pursuing and turn to other diagnostic possibilities. Put in terms of thresholds, this negative test result has moved you from above to below the 'test threshold' and you won't do any more tests for that diagnostic possibility. On the other hand, if the diagnostic test came back positive or generated a high likelihood ratio, the post-test probability might become so high that you would also abandon further testing because you'd made your diagnosis and would now move to choosing the most appropriate therapy; in these terms, you've now crossed from below to above the 'treatment threshold'. It's only if your diagnostic test result leaves you stranded between the test and treatment thresholds that you'd continue to pursue that initial diagnosis by performing other tests. Although there are some very fancy ways of calculating test and treatment thresholds from test accuracy and the risks and benefits of correct and incorrect

diagnostic conclusions,* intuitive test–treatment thresholds are commonly used by experienced clinicians and are another example of individual clinical expertise.

You may not cross a test–treatment threshold until you've performed several different diagnostic tests and here is where another nice property of the likelihood ratio comes into play. Because the post-test odds for the first diagnostic test you apply are the pretest odds for your second diagnostic test, you needn't switch back and forth between odds and probabilities between tests. You can simply keep multiplying the running product by the likelihood ratio generated from the next test. For example, when a 45-year-old man walks into your office his pretest probability of $\geq 75\%$ stenosis of one or more of his coronary arteries is about 6%. Suppose that he gives you a history of atypical chest pain (only two of the three symptoms of substernal chest discomfort, brought on by exertion, and relieved in <10 minutes by rest; a likelihood ratio of about 13) and that his exercise ECG reveals 2.2 mm of non-sloping ST-segment depression (a likelihood ratio of about 11). Then his post-test probability for coronary stenosis is his pretest probability [converted into odds] times the product of the likelihood ratios generated from his history (13) and exercise ECG (11), with the resulting post-test odds converted back to probabilities (through dividing by its value + 1): $(0.06 / 0.94) \times 13 \times 11 = 9.13 / 10.13 = 90\%$. The final result of these calculations is strictly accurate as long as the diagnostic tests being combined are 'independent' (that is, the probability of a specific result on the second is the same for any result on the first) and we know intuitively that this is not true for most of the diagnostic tests we apply in sequences aiming toward a single diagnosis. Accordingly, we'd want the calculated post-test probability at the end of this sequence to be comfortably above our treatment threshold before we would act upon it. This additional example of how likelihood ratios make lots of implicit diagnostic reasoning explicit is another argument in favor of generating overall

---

* See the recommendations for further reading or N Engl J Med 1980; 302: 1109.

likelihood ratios for sequences or clusters of diagnostic tests, as suggested back in Section 3b1.

We hope that you involved your patient as you worked your way through all the foregoing considerations that lead you to think that the diagnostic test is worth considering. If you haven't, you certainly need to do so now. Every diagnostic test involves some invasion of privacy and some are embarrassing, painful or dangerous. You'll have to be sure that the patient is an informed, willing partner in the undertaking. Finally, the ultimate question to ask about using any diagnostic test is whether its consequences (reassurance when negative, labeling and possibly generating awful diagnostic and prognostic news if positive, leading to further diagnostic tests and treatments, etc.) will help your patient achieve their goals of therapy. Included here are considerations of how subsequent interventions match clinical guidelines or restrictions on access to therapy designed to optimize the use of finite resources for all members of your society.

Further reading

Jaeschke R, Guyatt G H, Sackett D L for the Evidence-Based Medicine Working Group. Users' guides to the medical literature. VI. How to use an article about a diagnostic test. B. What are the results and will they help me in caring for my patients? JAMA 1994; 271: 703–7.

Section 4.2

Can you apply this valid, important evidence about prognosis in caring for your patient?

Having decided that the evidence you tracked down about prognosis is both valid and important, you now can consider how to use it in your clinical practice. Two guides can help you make these judgments; they appear in Table 4.2.1 and will be considered here.

First, were the study patients sufficiently similar to your own? The first guide asks you to compare your patients to those in the article and since presumably you know your patients well, this means trying to get to know the study patients well enough to compare them. Look for descriptions of the study sample, including the patients' demographics and important clinical characteristics. The more the study patients are like your patients, the more readily you can apply the results to your patients. Inevitably, some differences will turn up, so how similar is similar enough? To help you with this judgment, as in other places in this book, we suggest that you try this question framed the other way: are the study patients so different from yours that you'd expect their outcomes to be so different that they wouldn't be any use to you in making prognostic predictions about your patients?

Second, will this evidence make a clinically important impact on your conclusions about what to offer or tell your patient? If the evidence suggests a good prognosis when patients (especially in the early stages of disease) remain

Table 4.2.1 Can you apply this valid, important evidence about prognosis in caring for your patient?

1. Were the study patients similar to your own?
2. Will this evidence make a clinically important impact on your conclusions about what to offer or tell your patient?

untreated, that could strongly influence your discussion of treatment options with them. If, on the other hand, prognostic information derived from a control group in a randomized trial suggests a gloomy prognosis when no definitive therapy is instituted, your message to your patient would reflect this fact. And even when the prognostic evidence doesn't lead to a treat/don't treat decision, valid evidence is always useful in providing your patient or their family with the information they want to have about what the future is likely to hold for them and their illness.

Further reading

Laupacis A, Wells G, Richardson W S, Tugwell P for the Evidence-Based Medicine Working Group. Users' guides to the medical literature. V. How to use an article about prognosis. JAMA 1994; 272: 234–7.

Section 4.3

Can you apply this valid, important evidence about a treatment in caring for your patient?

In deciding whether valid, potentially useful results apply to your patient, you need once again to integrate the evidence with your clinical expertise. As shown in Table 4.3.1, there are two elements to this integration. The first estimates the impact of the treatment on patients just like yours and the second compares the values and preferences of your patient with the regimen and its consequences.

Estimating the impact of a valid, important treatment result on an individual patient

This element poses two additional questions: Do these results apply to your patient? How great would the potential benefit of therapy actually be for your individual patient?

Do these results apply to your patient?

Your patient wasn't in the trial that established the efficacy of this treatment. Maybe (because of their age, sex, comorbidity, disease severity or for a host of other sociodemographic, biologic or clinical reasons) they wouldn't even have been eligible for the trial. How can you extrapolate* from the external evidence to your individual patient? Rather than slavishly asking: 'Would my patient satisfy the eligibility criteria for the trial?' and rejecting its usefulness if they didn't exactly fit every one of them, we'd suggest bringing in some of your knowledge of human biology and

---

* Some teachers call this 'generalizing' from the trial, but really it's 'particularizing' to an individual patient, not generalizing to all patients, everywhere. Accordingly, we'll use the more generic term 'extrapolating'.

Table 4.3.1 Are these valid, potentially useful results applicable to your patient?

1. Do these results apply to your patient?
   ● Is your patient so different from those in the trial that its results can't help you?
   ● How great would the potential benefit of therapy actually be for your individual patient?
2. Are your patient's values and preferences satisfied by the regimen and its consequences?
   ● Do your patient and you have a clear assessment of their values and preferences?
   ● Are they met by this regimen and its consequences?

Table 4.3.2 Should you believe apparent qualitative differences in the efficacy of therapy in some subgroups of patients?

Only if you can say 'yes' to all of the following:
1. Does it really make biologic and clinical sense?
2. Is the qualitative difference both clinically (beneficial for some but useless or harmful for others) and statistically significant?
3. Was it hypothesized before the study began (rather than the product of dredging the data) and has it been confirmed in other, independent studies?
4. Was it one of just a few subgroup analyses carried out in this study?

clinical experience, turning the question around and asking: 'Is my patient so different from those in the trial that its results cannot help me make my treatment decision?' Pharmacogenetics aside, there are very few situations in which you would expect a drug or diet or operation to produce qualitatively different results in patients inside a trial and those who don't quite fit its eligibility criteria. Only if you conclude that your patient is so different from those in the study that its results simply don't inform your treatment decision should you discard its results.

What about subgroups?

Sometimes treatments appear to benefit some subgroups of patients but not others. For example, some of the early trials of aspirin for transient ischemic attacks suggested that this drug was efficacious in men but not in women. As is usually the case, this 'qualitative' difference in the effects of therapy (helpful for one group but useless or harmful in another) was a chance finding and later trials and overviews confirmed that aspirin is efficacious in women. The results from megatrials and overviews suggest that extrapolations from the overall results of individual trials usually are correct when applied to subgroups of patients in those trials. If you think that you may be dealing with one of the exceptions to this rule and that the treatment you're examining really does work in a qualitatively different way among

different patients, you should apply the guides in Table 4.3.2. In particular, unless this difference in response makes biologic sense, was hypothesized before the trial and has been confirmed in a second, independent trial, we'd suggest that you accept the treatment's overall efficacy as the best estimate of its efficacy in your patient.

So, unless there is some really powerful biologic reason for you to think that the treatment, if accepted by your patient, would be totally ineffectual or act in the opposing direction from the way it acted in patients in the study, we think you have good grounds for extrapolating the *direction* of the effect of the treatment on your patient's illness. Having decided that the direction of the treatment effect is likely to be the same as that observed in the study, you can now turn to considering whether that effect is likely to be great or small.

How great would the potential benefit of therapy be for your individual patient?

The trial report informed you about how the treatment worked in the average patient in the trial. How can you translate this to the probable treatment effect in your individual patient? We suggest that the measure we used to decide whether the treatment was potentially useful, the number of patients you need to treat (NNT) to prevent one bad outcome, is useful here. The trick is to translate the NNT

from the study into an NNT that fits your patient. You can do this the longer, harder (and maybe more accurate*) way or the quick and easy (but maybe less accurate) way.

The long way is to estimate the absolute susceptibility of your individual patient for developing the bad outcome over a period of time equal to the duration of the study. If the study you're using had a placebo or no-treatment group or subgroup with features like your patient, you could use their susceptibility† for this purpose. Another way would be to carry out a literature search to find a paper on the prognosis of patients like yours and use that figure. Either way, you'd take the resulting susceptibility (you could express it as a decimal fraction or a percentage, whichever you're more comfortable using) and multiply it by the RRR from the study. The result is the ARR and you can invert it to get the NNT. For example, if you find a prognosis paper suggesting that the susceptibility of your patient for a bad outcome is about 0.4 (the term we use to describe that susceptibility is the 'patient expected event rate' or PEER, so PEER = 40%) over a period of time equal to the duration of the trial that generated an RRR of 50%. Assuming that this RRR applies regardless of the susceptibility of patients in that trial, the ARR is PEER × RRR = 40% × 50% = 20% and the corresponding NNT is 1/ARR = 1/20% = 5 and you'd need to treat just five patients like yours for that length of time to prevent one event. If you would like to avoid these calculations, you can use the nomogram that appears in Figure 4.3.1. But there is an even easier way to estimate an NNT for patients like yours.

As we stated in the previous chapter, one of the reasons why the NNT is useful when interpreting the results of treatment trials is the ease with which it can be extrapolated to your own practice and to individual patients outside the trials. Through some very simple arithmetic, you can estimate NNTs for specific patients. All you need do is estimate the

* We're not being cute here. We all are pretty new at this and really don't know!
† Some people, especially when they use a control group to estimate susceptibility, call it 'baseline risk'.

susceptibility of your individual patient (if they were to receive just the control treatment) relative to the average control patient in the reported trial and convert this estimate into a decimal fraction we'll call F (if you judge your patient to be twice as susceptible as those in the trial, F = 2; if your patient is only half as susceptible as the average control patient in the trial, F = 0.5, and if just like the patients in the trial, F = 1). As long as the treatment produces a constant relative risk reduction across the spectrum of susceptibilities,* the NNT for your patient is simply the reported NNT divided by F. Going back to our intensive insulin example in Section 3b3, we learned that a group of clinical investigators had to treat 15 diabetics with intensive insulin regimens for 6.5 years in order to prevent one of them from developing diabetic neuropathy (NNT=15). If you judge that your patient was only half as susceptible as patients in that trial, F = 0.5 and NNT/F = 15/0.5 = 30, so 30 of these less susceptible patients would need to be treated for about 6.5 years with the intensive insulin regimen to prevent one of them from going on to develop neuropathy.

Comparing the values and preferences of your patient with the regimen and its consequences

A return to Table 4.3.1 identifies the steps to be taken here. You and your patient need to achieve a clear assessment of their values and preferences and then determine whether they will be served by the regimen in question. Sometimes the answer will be evident in a few seconds: for a patient having a heart attack, the value of survival and the preference for a simple, low-risk intervention like aspirin, given the efficacy of this regimen, usually makes this decision quickly agreed and acted upon. Other times the answer will take weeks and several visits to sort out: radiation or

* This is a big assumption and we're only beginning to learn when assuming a constant RRR is appropriate (for lots of medical treatments like antihypertensive drugs) and inappropriate (for some operations like carotid endarterectomy, where the RRR rises with increasing susceptibility).

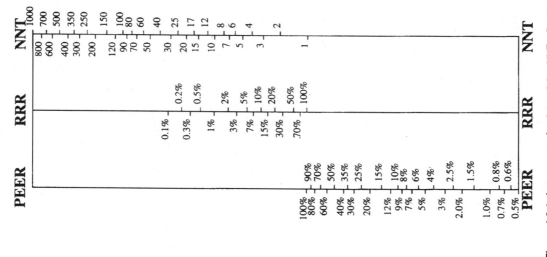

Figure 4.3.1 A nomogram for determining NNTs. Reprinted with permission from Chatellier G et al. The number needed to treat: a clinically useful nomogram in its proper context. BMJ 1996; 312: 426–9.

adjuvant chemotherapy for stage II carcinoma of the breast or transurethral resection of the prostate for moderate symptoms of prostatism.

Section 4.4

Can you apply this valid, important evidence about harm in caring for your patient?

In deciding whether and how to apply valid, potentially important results of a critical appraisal about a harmful treatment to an individual patient, four aspects of individual clinical expertise are important and they are listed in Table 4.4.1.

First, you need to decide whether the results of your critical appraisal can be extrapolated to your patient. As before, the issue is not whether your patient would have met all the inclusion criteria for the systematic review or individual study that demonstrated the harmful effect of the treatment, but whether your patient is so different from those in the report that its results provide no useful guidance for you.

Second, you need to estimate your patient's risk of the adverse outcome relative to the patients in the report. As we described in Section 4.3, if you can express this as a decimal fraction we'll call F (if your patient is twice the risk of those in the report, F=2; if half the risk, F=0.5; if the same risk, F=1) you can then simply divide the number of patients needed to be treated to produce one episode of harm (NNH) from the report by F. If, for example, you decided that a patient you're considering placing on an NSAID is at four times the risk of an upper GI bleed as those in a cohort study

that generated an NNH of 2000, the appropriate NNH for your patient becomes 2000/4 = 500.

Third, as with all clinical decisions, you need to identify and incorporate your patient's preferences, concerns and expectations into your recommendation. If they are 'risk-averse', on the one hand, or willing to gamble side-effects to gain possible treatment benefit, on the other, your discussions of the risks and benefits of the same treatment, even among patients with identical NNHs, may lead to very different treatment plans. At this point you can further modify NNH (or its F, whichever you are more comfortable dealing with) to take into account both your own and your patient's thoughts about the comparative health impacts of the treatment's adverse effect and the clinical event it was being used to prevent in the first place (represented by its NNT). If your patient is risk averse or if either of you thinks that the treatment's adverse effect (e.g. an intracranial bleed from anticoagulants) is 2–3 times as severe as the event the treatment was intended to prevent (recurrent deep vein thrombosis), you could double or triple the F for the NNH (or cut the NNH by 1/2 or 2/3) and then see how it compares with the NNT. If, on the other hand, your patient is a risk taker or the adverse treatment effect (e.g. cough from an ACE inhibitor) was only 1% as severe as the event the treatment was intended to prevent (death from heart failure), you could reduce the F for the NNH to 0.01 or multiply the NNH by 100.* In either case, the comparison of the treatment's 'adjusted' NNH with its NNT becomes very informative. If a treatment's NNH, after all this adjustment, is lower than its NNT, shouldn't you be considering some therapeutic alternatives? If your time and resources permit, this would be an ideal situation in which to carry out a clinical decision analysis.

Even if the adjusted NNH exceeds the NNT, you still ought to identify the possible alternative treatments (including no treatment!) you could offer your patient instead of the one

that produces this adverse effect. If a patient experienced wheezing when their hypertension was treated with a beta-blocker, it is easy to substitute another antihypertensive drug that is free of this side-effect. On the other hand, the alternatives to oral contraceptives for temporary conception control may not be acceptable to your patient, despite the small but real risk of thromboembolism from these drugs.

Further reading

Levine M, Walter S D, Lee H, Haines T, Holbrook A, Moyer V for the Evidence-Based Medicine Working Group. Users' guides to the medical literature. IV. How to use an article about harm. JAMA 1994; 271: 1615–19.

* In similar fashion, when a treatment (e.g. NSAIDs for arthritis) causes multiple adverse effects, you would apply a smaller F (or higher NNH) for a minor one (e.g. indigestion) than a major one (e.g. GI hemorrhage).

Table 4.4.1 Should these valid, potentially important results of a critical appraisal about a harmful drug change the treatment of an individual patient?

1. Can the study results be extrapolated to this patient?
2. What are this patient's risks of the adverse outcome?
3. What are this patient's preferences, concerns and expectations from this treatment?
4. What alternative treatments are available?

Section 4.6

Teaching methods relevant to the clinical application of the results of critical appraisals to individual patients

In this section we will present some strategies and tactics for teaching learners how to apply the results of their critical appraisals to patients. Because EBM begins and ends with patients, it is natural for us to use patient encounters for closing this loop. The message here is that critical appraisal and other elements of EBM are integral components of the everyday bedside and other clinical discussions of how to diagnose and manage patients and not peripheral topics to be discussed at other places and only when time permits. We will start with some obvious clinical situations, but then move progressively farther afield to demonstrate that closely similar strategies and tactics can be applied to a wide variety of teaching and learning situations. Finally, we will describe how several centers and academic consortia around the world operate 5-day workshops on how to practice EBM.

Working rounds on individual patients

First we will consider the 'working round' in which a clinical team review the problems and progress of patients on a clinical service or in an outpatient setting. These are held in various formats. On an inpatient unit, they might consist of a walking round in which every patient on the service is briefly presented, seen and discussed. In an outpatient setting, they might focus on a single patient who has been asked to stay behind or might consider the entire session's patients after they've left. Finally, they might be quite informal gatherings over coffee in which discussions around patients are tagged onto meetings that deal largely with administrative and housekeeping tasks. When the available time is in harmony with the numbers of patients to be seen

(or at least discussed), these can provide excellent opportunities for teaching and learning EBM. Often, however, time is short and the list of patients long and in those circumstances many services adopt a two-stage approach in which they begin by sitting down and quickly reviewing the patient list and then focus on just those patients in whom major decisions have to be made. In either format, patients are presented (and, if available, examined), followed by discussions in which management decisions are taken and defended with the best available evidence. How might these discussions be organized to maximize the opportunities for learning and practicing EBM? Two tactics are useful here.

The first ties EBM to the presentation of the patient. Back in Chapter 1 we described how the educational prescription could be used to initiate finding and critically appraising evidence and in Table 1.5 we showed how it could form the final element in presenting a new patient. In a similar fashion, as shown in Table 4.6.1, filling that educational Rx can form the final element of presenting a patient already known to the clinical service. In this fashion, the scientific justification for a diagnostic or therapeutic course of action becomes part of describing the past and planning the future care of the patient and serves the decision-making as well as educational requirements of the meeting.

The second tactic concerns the actual presentation of the evidence. The busier the service, the more important that evidence central to management decisions is concisely and quickly presented. This is where the CATs (introduced back in Section 3b7) can come in so handy.* After hearing about and (if possible) examining the patient, the team can gather around the resulting CAT, quickly decide whether its clinical bottom line applies, make the management decision and get on to the next patient (requesting copies of CATs for further study or later use).

* For greatest effect, CATs have to be produced in real time while decisions are being made (often easier between visits in ambulatory settings than overnight in inpatient settings). To speed their production, a CAT-Maker is available on disk or via the Website at the Oxford Centre for Evidence-Based Medicine (http://cebm.jr2.ox.ac.uk/).

Table 4.6.1 A guide for learners in presenting an 'OLD'* patient at follow-up rounds

The presentation should summarize 20 things in less than 2 minutes:

1. The patient's surname.
2. Their age.
3. Their gender.
4. Their occupation/social role.
5. When they were admitted.
6. Their chief complaint(s) that led directly to their admission.
7. The number of ACTIVE PROBLEMS that they have at the present time.
   And then, for each ACTIVE PROBLEM (a problem could be a symptom, sign, event, diagnosis, injury, psychological state, social predicament, etc.):
8. Its most important symptoms, if any.
9. Its most important signs, if any.
10. The results of diagnostic or other exploratory/confirmatory investigations.
11. The explanation (diagnosis or state) for the problem.
12. The treatment plan instituted for the problem.
13. The response to this treatment plan.
14. The future plans for managing this problem. Repeat 8–14 for each ACTIVE PROBLEM.
15. Your plans for discharge, posthospital care and follow-up.
16. Whether you've filled the educational prescription that you requested when this patient was admitted (in order to better understand the patient's pathophysiology, clinical findings, diagnosis, prognosis, therapy, prevention of recurrence, quality of care or other important issue in order to become a better clinician). If so:
17. How you found the relevant evidence.
18. What you found. The clinical bottom line derived from that evidence.
19. Your critical appraisal of that evidence for its VALIDITY and APPLICABILITY.
20. How that critically appraised evidence will alter your care of that (or the next similar) patient. If not, when you are going to fill it.

* That is, a patient already known to the service.

The sorts of words you might use:

A. Mr/Mrs/Ms/Prof/PC 11111 is a 22222 year-old 33333 44444 who was admitted on 55555 with the chief complaint of 66666.
B. They have 77777 Active Problems.
C. The first active problem is _____
It is characterized by 88888 and 99999 and we _____ which revealed 10-10-10.
We decided that the cause for this problem was _____ performed a
11-11-11-11 and we started 12-12-12-12, to which he/she responded with 13-13-13-13. We plan to 14-14-14-14.
D. The second/third/fourth active problem is _____ (repeat 8-14)
E. At the time of her/his admission, I didn't understand _____ as well as I'd like to and I requested an educational Rx to answer the question: _____

I found the relevant evidence by 17-17-17-17 and its clinical bottom line is 18-18-18-18. I believe that this bottom line is/is not valid because 19a-19a-19a-19a and I believe that it is/is not applicable because 19b-19b-19b. I therefore plan to manage this and future, similar patients by 20-20-20-20.

Small groups and 'academic half-days'

Quite often, learners from different clinical teams gather at regularly scheduled educational sessions to receive general instruction in the evaluation and management of patients. The numbers of learners at these sessions can range from a handfull to a hall-full and running them on a 'set-piece' lecture format can tax the ability of the teachers to stay enthused and the ability of the learners to stay awake. An alternative approach builds on the self-directed, problem-based EBM learning orientation and runs as follows:

1. Learners are asked to identify clinical problems for which they are uncertain about the best way to diagnose or manage affected patients (stating their uncertainties in the form of clinical questions, as in Chapter 1, specifying the patient, the intervention and the outcome of interest to them). Training programs employing this approach report a distinct

pattern in the problems that learners identify. Early on, post-graduates identify medical emergencies in which they are unsure of their skills at diagnosing and managing life-threatening situations. Many programs anticipate these concerns and have basic and advanced cardiac and/or trauma support training at the ready.

2. Once the foregoing concerns are addressed, postgraduates identify a wide array of management problems in which they are not sure how to treat patients with specific disorders, followed by clinical problems in diagnosis, prognosis and etiology (especially for iatrogenic disorders). Occasionally, interest is expressed in a locally occurring quality of care study or audit, in their own continuing education, and in health economics. When several learners identify the same clinical situation,* it joins the schedule for a future session and the following processes occur:

● Acting in rotation, one or more of the learners takes on the task of searching the clinical literature for valid, relevant systematic reviews or primary articles on the clinical problem. Along the way, with help from librarians as needed, they develop and hone their skills in searching for the best evidence.

● With faculty guidance, they pick the one or two articles of highest validity and relevance and these, along with a description of the clinical problem, are copied and distributed to everyone to be studied in advance of the session.

● At that session, and again with faculty guidance as needed, they lead the discussion of the validity and potential usefulness of the evidence presented in the paper. Presenters often aid the discussion by introducing CATs or other summaries and displays of the most relevant evidence. This critical appraisal is integrated with discussions of the related pathophysiology and clinical skills, with the final objective of generating a common, evidence-based approach to the clinical

---

* Part of an initial session can be devoted to reaching consensus on priority clinical problems and such discussions can be repeated as current topics are exhausted and new topics arise.

problem. In some cases, the learners may want to work with senior clinicians to generate and circulate their own guidelines for future use.

Over the years, teachers of EBM have discovered lots of ways *not* to teach effectively and several ways that seem to work. We have summarized them in the form of a set of teaching tips, which appear in Table 4.6.2.

Journal clubs

Journal clubs are dying or dead in many clinical centers, especially when they rely on a rota through which members are asked to summarize the latest issues of preassigned journals. When you think about it, that sort of journal club is run by the postman, not the clinicians or patients, and it is no wonder that it is becoming extinct. On the other hand, a few journal clubs are flourishing and a growing number of them are designed and conducted along EBM lines. They operate like the 'academic half-days' described above.

Each meeting of the journal club has three parts:

1. In one part, journal club members describe patients who exemplify clinical situations which they are uncertain how best to diagnose or manage. This discussion continues until there is consensus that a particular clinical problem,* which we'll call problem C, is worth the time and effort necessary to find its solution. Then either the member who nominated the problem or another member, based on a rota, takes responsibility for performing a search for the best evidence on problem C.

2. In a second part, the results of the evidence search on last session's problem (we'll call it problem B) are shared in the form of photocopies of the abstracts of 4–6 systematic reviews, original articles or other evidence. Club members decide which one or two pieces of evidence are worth studying and arrangements are made to get copies of the clinical problem statement and best evidence to all members well in advance of the next meeting.

---

* Stated (as in Chapter 1) in terms of a patient, an intervention (and a comparison intervention if appropriate) and an outcome.

Table 4.6.2 Some teaching tips for EBM*

Motivating learning

A. Keep the session relevant and meaningful to learners.

1. Select (or help them track down) articles that relate to patients in their care and pick 'good' articles. Types of good articles for critical appraisal purposes (in decreasing order of their liveliness potential) include those that provide:
   - ground-breaking but solid evidence at the forefront of clinical practice (especially if not yet in widespread use);
   - solid evidence that a common practice is worthless;
   - solid evidence that a common practice ought to be questioned;
   - for common or controversial practices:
     (i) a pair of articles – a bad one to trash, maybe after reading no further than the methods, plus a good one to use for decision making or,
     (ii) a bad article with high trash titres but nonetheless the best one available;
   - NOTE: solid evidence supporting current practice is an excellent place to start (so as to avoid cynicism or nihilism) but risks boring more experienced learners.

2. Start sessions with a patient's problem (real or simulated) and end sessions by coming to a conclusion about how to manage the patient.

3. Save time for closure. Come to closure about both the article and the patient. Closure does not necessarily require unanimous agreement. The group may agree that the evidence is fairly solid but still not agree on individuals' decisions for the patient in the scenario.

4. If a methodological issue comes up that may sidetrack the discussion, ask the group how they want to handle it (usually it can be deferred and discussed with just the subset of learners who are interested in deeper methodology).

B. Keep the learners active.

1. Ask the learners to vote on what they would do clinically before the article is discussed. Ask them to write down their recommendations and pass in their scripts anonymously to avoid embarrassment.

2. When someone asks a question, NEVER ridicule them.

3. Turn questions back to the person asking or to the entire group: 'What does the group think?', 'Can anyone help out here?'

4. Call on people only when they feel comfortable and know it is 'OK' not to know.

5. Ask challenging (but not intimidating) open-ended questions. 'What do the authors mean by a randomized trial?' vs 'Is this a randomized trial?'

6. When bias might be present in an article, ask the group to decide if it might be important. If present, in what direction would it influence the results, i.e. would it widen or narrow a difference between groups? Do a worst case scenario analysis. Would this bias, if present and affecting all members of a group, reverse the analysis? (In other words, could this bias be a fatal flaw?)

7. When discussing diagnostic tests, go right to likelihood ratios (omit sensitivity, specificity, prevalence, etc.), go straight to the relevant 2×2 table and help the learners generate the appropriate proportions and calculations, asking them as you go along to express what the calculations mean in words. Only afterwards ask them to put names to these concepts, like sensitivity, specificity, etc.*

8. Summarize specific points during the session; check if it's OK to move on to the next topic. Stop from time to time to synthesize and summarize to show the group that there is a set of take-home messages even though full closure may not have occurred.

9. Time out: when particular problems or successes are occurring in the group dynamic, call 'time out' to divert attention to the group process rather than the clinical problem. Examine with the group what is occurring in the interaction, then call 'time in' to return to the clinical problem. Time outs can be especially useful when the teacher senses tension: call a time out, tell the group you sense tension and ask them what's going on.

C. Show your enthusiasm for critical appraisal in general and look for opportunities to compliment your specific set of learners and the work they are doing.

D. Novelty (once your team become adept at critical appraisal).

1. Use more controversial clinical topics and articles.

2. Use articles that come to different conclusions on the same topic.

3. In non-clinical situations, use 'role play' and scenarios. For role play, if people are reluctant, ask them to just play themselves, in the situations they find in their daily work life. Other situations to try include: courtrooms and malpractice claims, formal debates, point-counterpoint (appoint individuals to each role), hostile residents (or consultants!) on teaching rounds.

4. Introduce a 'quick challenge' or 'snap diagnosis' for an article with a fatal flaw, especially if you sense or discover that the group has not prepared in advance, start the session with: 'Quick, is there a fatal flaw in this paper and if so, what is it?'

Learning climate

A. Learners must feel comfortable identifying and addressing their limitations.

1. Be open about your own limitations and the things you don't know.

2. Use educational prescriptions (see page 33).

3. Periodically, make it a point to say that no one knows everything and that is why we are all here.

4. Encourage people to ask questions.

5. Have fun.

6. Provide feedback. Nod your head or make some reinforcing comment, especially when a correct response is given to a question or someone brings up an important issue.

B. Fight 'critical appraisal nihilism' ('No study is perfect, so what good is any of the literature?').

1. Select good articles, especially at the start.

2. Put the article into perspective in terms of what is known in the research area. This may be the first clinical trial of a new treatment.

3. Ask learners what they would look for in (or, if they are keen to do research, how they would design) a better study on this clinical issue.

4. Remind the learners that they have to use what is available in the literature for clinical decision making. Application of critical appraisal to clinical decision making is a positive process; not using critical appraisal can result in mindless adoption of faulty practices. Mindlessness is more nihilistic than questioning and seeking the right answer.

5. Separate innocent and possible problems from fatal flaws.

6. Help learners sort the literature and the clinical practice it supports into three categories: definitely useful, incompletely tested and definitely useless.

7. Remind the learners that it may be the editors' and not the authors' fault that insufficient information is provided in the published article.

*Credit for the original compilation of this list goes to Martha Gerrity and Valerie Lawrence.

* Like lots of the elements of EBM, these concepts are not difficult but their jargon can be mystifying, so if you can orient students to the numbers and get them to say what they mean, you can later apply the usual terms, hopefully now demystified.

C. How to handle statistics.

1. Note the difference between statistical significance and clinical importance.
2. Use the 'statistics isn't important' technique. As a tutor, don't permit the session to turn into an attempt to teach statistics. Tell group members that study methods, samples, clinical measurements, follow-up and clinical conclusions are what's important and that statistics are merely tools to help these processes. If good methods were used, the investigators probably went to the effort to use good statistics (the 'trust 'em' mode). If bad methods were used, good statistics could never rescue the study (garbage in/garbage out, the frog is a frog and not a prince).
3. Suggest the quick and dirty sample size calculations such as the inverse rule of 3 on page 107.

Group control of the session

A. Discuss the goals of the session at its beginning and check along the way on whether it's making progress, especially if the discussion seems to be getting off track.

B. Learners' agenda versus teacher's agenda.

1. Try to go with the learners' agenda as much as possible. They will not learn all there is to know about critical appraisal in one session – remember how long it took you to learn it.
2. Let the group generate their own agenda for a specific session. This may lead into uncharted territory but learning will often be increased. The unlikely outcome is that closure may not be achieved, so be on guard to reassure (and, if you can't stand the chaos, provide direction).
3. Evaluate at the end to see if all goals were accomplished and how the next session could be more productive, more learner centered, more active, more stimulating and more fun.

C. When individuals try to dominate the discussion, put down others or 'know it all', take a 'time out' and ask the group to discuss individual responsibilities to the group. This should facilitate discussion of individual responsibilities and provide energy for individuals to take more responsibility (by the loud ones lightening up and the quiet ones contributing more).

D. When individuals or the whole group clam up and won't participate (not unusual at the first session).

1. Wait the 'magic 17 seconds'. No one can stand silence for more than about 5 seconds and the tutor who knows

(and believes!) this can outwait any group or member, no matter how long it takes. Refrain from jumping in to fill the silence yourself or they'll know that they don't have to take responsibility for their learning.

2. Take a 'time out' and ask the group members to discuss individual responsibilities to the group in terms of participation.
3. A possible script of questions to get a clinical problem + clinical article session going:
● How should we manage this clinical problem?
● What was there about the clinical article that supports that clinical decision (if unanimous) or those different decisions (if group members disagree on management)?
● (At this point it often becomes clear that some, and maybe all, group members haven't read the article). Does anybody need time to scan the article? (If so, you may want to give them 5 minutes to see what they can glean from it.) Alternatively, you could ask them to identify the features of an article that would be most helpful to them, then assign paragraphs of the methods section to pairs of learners and have them report back to the group on how well the article met their information needs.
● In the subsequent discussion, tease out and label the critical appraisal guides (emphasizing their generic importance rather than just how well they were met by the article).
● If the group is stalled, you could give them the guides, assigning one each to pairs of group members, have them work for a few minutes in pairs and report back to the group what they concluded and how it affects their clinical decision.
● What can we conclude and use in our clinical practice? Everyone agree?
● On which clinical issues did we achieve closure? On which not? See, lifelong learning is necessary!
4. Another question to foster discussion: The methods may be sound but are the results compelling? Concepts to bring out include statistical versus clinical significance, number needed to treat, etc.

E. Cures for the 'jumping around' or 'tangent' syndrome.

1. Remember that this syndrome is not always, or even usually, a disease. It regularly leads to long-lasting competencies in the areas under discussion, especially when the disparate elements are brought together by a skilled tutor.
2. Fill in the blank spaces on a blackboard (laid out with your mind's-eye framework of the relevant list of critical

appraisal guides) as the group comes up with and discusses the relevant issues. This will allow an unstructured discussion in which learners can generate criteria, points, etc. in any order that naturally arises, yet close with a coherent, ordered summary of the key guides and issues.

3. Check your watch frequently to see how the process is going. If a lot is being generated, don't worry about keeping a particular order or you'll risk stifling creativity and active learning.
4. Try to come up with 'segues' or transitional comments to tie what might appear to be tangential issues back into the clinical business at hand.

F. Capitalize on disagreements by asking for their bases in evidence or its critical appraisal. Where possible, reconcile them as arising from the application of different critical appraisal guides or from different interpretations of evidence related to the same guide. These reconciliations can be used to involve the rest of the group and to achieve closure on the particular issue.

G. When a learner asks a question directly to the tutor, allow the question to deflect onto another member of the tutorial, by pausing or by invitation. This can accomplish two things: (a) increase the group participation, and show them that they can teach each other, (b) buy time for you to think, in case the answer isn't immediately apparent to you but you don't want to admit that too soon!

Jargon

1. Explain a concept first, then label it with the jargon term. Better yet, get the group to explain the concept.
2. Ask learners who use jargon to explain the term to the rest of the group.

Finally

Remember that those learning to practice and teach EBM usually progress through two or three levels of expertise:

1. They become very good at sniffing out biases in articles (but don't yet know their consequences). They become highly critical and risk becoming entrenched nihilists.
2. They progress to being able to identify both the presence and direction of bias, so that they can sort out whether it's tending to produce false-positive or false-negative conclusions (and can be reassured when the latter makes a positive conclusion even more, rather than less, clinically relevant). They are ready for at least intuitive sensitivity analyses. You'd like your learners to get at least this far by the end of their training.

3. The main part of the journal club session is spent in a discussion critically appraising the evidence found in response to the clinical problem the club identified two sessions ago (we'll call it problem A) and about which it selected evidence for detailed study one session ago. The evidence is critically appraised for its validity and applicability and a decision made about whether and how it could be applied to future patients cared for by members of the journal club. This is the 'pay-off' part of the session and every effort should be made to ensure that 'closure' is reached. Ideally, a CAT is generated along the way, for discussion, revision and distribution to all the journal club members.

The actual order of these three parts of the journal club meeting could be reversed, depending on local preferences and tardiness!

Grand rounds and clinical conferences

Most hospitals hold weekly sessions in the auditorium for either their entire clinical staff or one of its departments. These sessions, which go by different names in different places, are conducted in order to discuss health issues of common interest and to try to accomplish continuing education and continuing professional development. They vary enormously in their subject matter (from molecular medicine to health reform) and in the passivity of their audience and in many hospitals patients have long since disappeared from the scene.

A common thread is the attempt to instruct the audience and transfer facts to them. Alas, as we learned back in the

Introduction, such instructional forms of CME, although they may increase knowledge, don't on average bring about either useful changes in clinical behavior or improvements in the quality of care.

Could a return to the grand round of a former era improve the situation? Building on that tradition and emphasizing some principles of EBM, these meetings could take on a different flavor and convert the audience from passive to active mode. The tactics are the following:

1. The rounds begin by focusing on a specific individual patient in the care of the presenters and the patient (whenever possible), images of the patient and undigested clinical data about the patient are presented.

2. The audience are required to assess this evidence, to generate opinions on its normalcy and diagnostic, prognostic or therapeutic implications and to report their individual opinions to the assembly by show of hands. To eliminate embarrassment and encourage participation, this reporting can be done anonymously by ticking diagnostic forms and then executing two or three exchanges among neighbors so that subsequent shows of hands are known not to represent the reporter's own opinion.* Of course, this solution is unnecessary in lecture halls equipped with anonymous, keypad voting systems.

3. A critical appraisal of the relevant evidence on the case is presented in an interactive fashion, requiring the audience to offer opinions on its validity and applicability.

4. A hand-out is provided at the end of the round, summarizing both the relevant evidence and the critical appraisal guides for determining its validity and clinical applicability. In this fashion, an actively participating audience not only take stands on the appropriate evaluation and management of a real patient, but also receive a carry-away reinforcement

* It works! The author has used this approach over 100 times, with clinical audiences from five continents, and reckons that it produces participation rates of over 80%. A videotape of such a round (Clinical Disagreement about a Patient with Dysphagia) is available from the Centre for Evidence-Based Medicine in Oxford.

and set of guides that they can apply in other, similar situations.

Lectures (for preclinical students and clinicians of all ages and stages)

This entry may appear to be out of place! How could lectures, especially for preclinical students with no clinical skills or clinical judgment, focus in an active, interactive fashion on the care of individual patients? Well, they can, based on two realizations. First, even first year premedical students already have life experiences of a wide array of illnesses: all fear contracting AIDS, most have a relative with symptomatic coronary heart disease and many know someone with breast cancer. On the first day of school, they possess an array of personal clinical examples from which to consider the entire range of EBM topics. Second, there are unorthodox ways of employing lecture halls filled with students in ways that encourage active learning around EBM. This is perhaps best introduced by an example and the one that we will employ is a lecture to a first-year premedical class in biostatistics and epidemiology at Oxford.*

1. A clinical scenario is presented (on overheads), describing the clinical history and physical examination of a patient the speaker was called to see in an emergency room (in brief, a man who smells of alcohol and feces comes in complaining of a rapidly enlarging abdomen).

2. The students are asked to form pairs and write down the two most important facts they've been given about the patient and the two most likely explanations for his presentation. The lecturer then leaves the room for 5 minutes.

3. On return (to the sound of 60 active discussions!), the students report back their judgments and it quickly becomes apparent that there is remarkable preclinical consensus on what are considered 'clinical' issues of diagnosis.

* A videotape of this lecture (A Stercoraceous Man with a Swollen Abdomen) is available from the Centre for Evidence-Based Medicine in Oxford.

Evidence-based Medicine

4. The students are then asked to identify the next most useful bit of evidence about their diagnostic explanations and the ensuing discussion around the precision and accuracy of clinical signs and symptoms introduces sensitivity, specificity, pre- and post-test probabilities, likelihood ratios and the like for later use by the faculty teaching the rest of the course.

5. Once the diagnosis and initial treatment are discussed, the issue of long-term management arises and a journal article reporting a randomized trial is distributed. Students are asked to form quartets in order to take and defend stands on whether the treatment advocated in this report should be offered to the patient. The lecturer then leaves the room for 10 minutes.

6. On return (to the roar of 30 therapeutic debates!), the students again report back their judgments and why they've decided to accept or reject the therapeutic recommendations in the published paper. The discussion introduces another host of methodological topics around descriptive and inferential statistics, statistical significance, clinically useful measures of efficacy and other topics for later use by the faculty throughout the rest of the course.

The other teachers in this course kept coming back to this patient example as they introduced the principles and methods of epidemiology and biostatistics. The students reported (in addition to enjoyment) the growing realization of the manifest relevance of understanding some epidemiological and biostatistical methodology to their goals of becoming effective clinicians.

Workshops on how to practice EBM

Although clinical learners can and do acquire the skills and knowledge for practicing EBM 'on the job' as they proceed through their careers (and this is the only site where they learn how to integrate external evidence with individual clinical expertise and apply the synthesis to patients), many learners also seek opportunities for more concentrated and focused education in its critical appraisal components. For the last 15 years, such opportunities have been provided in

the form of workshops of a few hours' to a few days' duration. Originated at McMaster University in Canada, the workshop format has spread to other centers and countries and has been organized by various academic and professional groups, including a group of UK medical students who, impatient with the pace of change in undergraduate medical education, organized and ran their own 5-day workshop!* These workshops have four elements in common.

First, the learning is problem based and is typically centered around clinical scenarios describing actual patients who have been in the care of one of the faculty, accompanied by relevant research evidence (usually from the clinical literature), and calling for the learners to generate and answer questions about the clinical situation. Initially, the external evidence is provided, but later it may be the result of searches performed by the participants. By the end of the workshop, the participants will be expected to begin to pose their own questions about their own patients. An example of a clinical scenario with its citation appears in Table 4.6.3 and similar 'packages' are prepared for each of the disciplines (medicine, surgery, general practice, etc.), addressing issues in diagnosis, prognosis, therapy, systematic reviews, harm, economic analysis and quality of care.

Second, learning tends to occur in small groups of 5–10 participants with one or two tutors/facilitators who are skilled in teaching EBM and in running small groups. This provides an environment that encourages active learning and often replicates the clinical team settings in which EBM will be practiced subsequently. While carefully avoiding behavioral therapy, these groups also instruct and encourage their members in more effective and efficient team function by developing and following rules such as those that appear in Table 4.6.4. Each group meeting begins by setting an agenda for the session (including setting aside time for breaks, evaluation, future planning); agreeing on the clinical problem, the roles of group members, the edu-

Table 4.6.3 A clinical scenario to initiate problem-based learning around an issue in therapy

You learn that a 54 y/o man with NIDDM (on oral hypoglycemics) whose myocardial infarction you treated 6 months ago has died suddenly at home. Wondering whether you could have done more for him, you review his notes and confirm that his was, in fact, a low-risk inferior MI with no complications whose blood sugar was elevated on admission (13 mmol/L) but settled down within 3 days.

In view of the success of 'tight control' of IDDM in preventing or postponing retinopathy and neuropathy, you wonder if a more aggressive treatment of his NIDDM might have postponed his untimely death. On the other hand, you well recall how one of your Profs back in medical school insisted that insulin was atherogenic and how you should back off insulin doses when diabetics developed angina pectoris.

So you form the clinical question: 'Among patients with NIDDM who are having MIs, does tight control of their blood sugar reduce their risk of dying?'

On your own or with help from the librarian at your local postgraduate center, you find the attached article: Malmberg K et al Randomized trial of insulin-glucose infusion followed by subcutaneous insulin treatment in diabetic patients with acute myocardial infarction (DIGAMI Study). J Am Coll Cardiol 1995; 26: 57–65.*

Read it (to possibly help you, we've included bits of a book on how to read clinical articles) and decide:
1. whether it answers your question;
2. if so, what the answer is,
whether you and your hospital colleagues should review how you are treating diabetic patients with myocardial infarctions.

* It can also be found on the disk version of ACP Journal Club/Evidence-Based Medicine or via MEDLINE using the terms: diabetes mellitus AND myocardial infarction AND publication type=randomized controlled trial.

cational tasks and the evidence to be appraised; getting on with it (calling 'time out' when either the process or the content is getting bogged down); evaluating this session;

* Named OCCAMS for Oxford Conference on Critical Appraisal for Medical Students and involving students from England, Scotland, Northern Ireland, Germany, Sweden and Croatia.

Table 4.6.5 A typical schedule for a workshop on how to practice EBM

Time	Sunday	Monday	Tuesday	Wednesday	Thursday	Friday
0800		Tutors' meetings				
0900		Plenary sessions on forming questions, searching, etc.				Small groups
1000		Small groups	Small groups	Small groups	Small groups	Small groups
1100						Evaluation
1200	Lunch					Good-bye
1300	Tutors' meeting	Individual study or ad hoc interest group meetings or individual searching				
1400						
1500						
1600		Small groups	Small groups	Small groups	Small groups	Small groups
1700		Small groups	Small groups	Small groups	Small groups	Small groups
1800	Supper					
Evening	Social	Study	Social	Study	Social	

Table 4.6.4 How small groups succeed in learning EBM (or anything else)

1. By taking responsibility (individually and as a group) for showing up and on time; by learning each other's names, interests and objectives; by respecting each other; by contributing to, accepting and supporting individual and group rules of behavior, including confidentiality; by contributing to, accepting and supporting both the overall objectives of the group and the detailed plans and assignments for each session; by carrying out the agreed plans and assignments, including role playing; by listening (concentrating and analyzing, rather than simply preparing your own response to what's being said) and by talking (including consolidating and summarizing).

2. By monitoring and (by using time in/time out*) reinforcing positive and correcting negative elements of both:
   - 'process', regarding educational methods (reinforcing positive contributions and teaching methods; proposing strategies for improving less effective ones) and responsibility (identifying behaviors, not motives; encouraging [e.g. with eye-contact, verbally] non-participants; quieting down [e.g. move them next to tutor] overparticipants); and
   - 'content': unclear, uncertain or incorrect facts or critical appraisal principles/ strategies/ tactics.

3. By evaluating selves, each other, the group, the session and the program with candour and respect, 'celebrating' what went well (and should be preserved) and identifying what went poorly, focusing on strategies for correcting/ improving the situation.

* Time in for the teaching/learning portions of the session, especially when using role play, time out for discussions of effective/ineffective teaching/learning methods and group/individual behavior.

and planning for the next one. Thus, the learning focuses on the five steps that form the major chapters of this book:

1. forming answerable questions;
2. searching for the best evidence (workshops usually include individual tutorials by librarians experienced in teaching searching skills);
3. critically appraising the evidence (the major focus of most workshops);
4. integrating the appraisal with individual clinical expertise and applying it in practice (this element can only be carried out when workshops are spread out over longer periods of time, with regular clinical responsibilities taking place between sessions); and
5. self-evaluation.

Given the foregoing, the selection of participants (in addition to responding to consumer demand and general interest) seeks individuals who are already receptive to EBM (skeptics make important contributions to workshops and are welcome additions to the converted) and are likely to be able to apply what they learn in their clinical practice. Most evaluations suggest that small groups made up of clinicians in the same discipline (e.g. general practice, surgery, nursing, etc.) learn best, as they can work on scenarios specific to their disciplines and more readily see how they might apply the results of their growing skills in practice. The exceptions to this rule are methodologists such as epidemiologists and biostatisticians, who are often used to functioning in disparate groups and can contribute to one of any make-up. The play of chance and small numbers (surgical specialities often are underrepresented) sometimes makes for unusual combinations of disciplines and these often require additional attention to be sure that alternative scenarios are presented to maintain relevance for all members.

Third, lots of time is set aside for small group meetings, individual study and meetings of ad hoc interest groups. Educational materials are sent out well in advance (with a reassurance that not all will have to be mastered before the workshop!). A typical schedule is shown in Table 4.6.5. Tutors meet daily to report progress, to make mid-course corrections in the workshop and to identify and solve problems in group function and learning (their training occurs in the 'how to teach EBM' workshops described in Chapter 5). Plenary sessions are kept to a minimum and deal only with issues best communicated in a lecture or lecture-audience participation format (a review of EBM, how to pose answerable questions, an introduction to information searching, etc.) and a final feedback and evaluation session where participants hand in their evaluation forms and suggest improvements for future workshops.

Some workshops are held in one-day or half-day sessions, spread out over longer periods of time. Less efficient for organizers, these often merge with the journal clubs described above and provide more opportunities for integrating the critical appraisals with individual clinical expertise as the EBM skills are acquired.

Fourth, participants and organizers keep in touch after the workshops in order to continue to trade ideas on how to practice EBM, how to improve future workshops and so that some of the participants can move to the next level of not only practicing EBM but teaching it as well. These workshops will be described in Chapter 5.

Further information

Get on the WWW and browse the educational resources of the Centre for Evidence-Based Medicine in Oxford by contacting the Uniform Resource Locator: http://cebm.jr2.ox.ac.uk/

Individuals interested in attending or organizing workshops in how to practise EBM can contact either the Department of Clinical Epidemiology and Biostatistics at McMaster University (1200 Main Street West, Hamilton, Ontario, Canada L8N 3Z5) or any of the Centres for Evidence-Based Practice in the UK (for example: http://cebm.jr2.ox.ac.uk/ will get you to the Website for the Centre for Evidence-Based Medicine in Oxford).